28 Days

What Your Cycle Reveals about Your Love Life, Moods, and Potential

Gabrielle Lichterman

Foreword by Scott Haltzman, M.D.

Polka Dot Press
Avon, Massachusetts

For my husband, Douglas.

Published by
Polka Dot Press, an imprint of
Adams Media, an F+W Publications Company
57 Littlefield Street, Avon, MA 02322. U.S.A.
www.adamsmedia.com

ISBN: 1-59337-345-7

Printed in Canada.

J I H G F E D C B A

Library of Congress Cataloging-in-Publication Data
Lichterman, Gabrielle.
28 days / Gabrielle Lichterman.
p.   cm.
ISBN 1-59337-345-7
1. Menstrual cycle—Popular works. 2. Menstrual cycle—
Psychological aspects—Popular works. I. Title: Twenty-eight days. II. Title.
QP263.L53 2005
612.6'62—dc22

2004026342

28 Days is intended as a reference volume only, not as a medical manual. In light
of the complex, individual, and specific nature of health problems, this book is not
intended to replace professional medical advice. The ideas, procedures, and suggestions in this book are intended to supplement, not replace, the advice of a trained
medical professional. Consult your physician before adopting the suggestions in this
book, as well as about any condition that may require diagnosis or medical attention.
The author and publisher disclaim any liability arising directly or indirectly from the
use of this book.

This publication is designed to provide accurate and authoritative information with
regard to the subject matter covered. It is sold with the understanding that the publisher is not engaged in rendering legal, accounting, or other professional advice.
If legal advice or other expert assistance is required, the services of a competent
professional person should be sought.
—From a *Declaration of Principles* jointly adopted by a Committee of the American Bar Association and a Committee of Publishers and Associations

Many of the designations used by manufacturers and sellers to distinguish their
products are claimed as trademarks. Where those designations appear in this book
and Adams Media was aware of a trademark claim, the designations have been
printed in initial capital letters.

This book is available at quantity discounts for bulk purchases.
For information, please call 1-800-872-5627.

Acknowledgments

A ginormous thank you to my agent, June Clark. Your guidance, wisdom, and patience are unrivaled.

A great big thanks to my editor, Danielle Chiotti, for her expertise and humor, and for recognizing the heart of this project.

I'd like to express my gratitude to Dr. Scott Haltzman, who supported this project from the beginning and was always there when I needed advice.

To my husband, Douglas, I am forever grateful for all the love, support, cheerleading, and home-brewed "book juice" that kept me researching and typing into the wee hours of the morning.

Finally, this project would not have been possible if it weren't for the many researchers who saw the wisdom in conducting studies on how hormones affect menstruating women's lives. Your work has been illuminating.

Day 1   Day 2   Day 3   Day 4   Day 5   Day 6   Day 7

Contents

Day 8   Day 9   Day 10   Day 11   Day 12   Day 13   Day 14

Foreword

Every single part of the body is connected to another. You sniffle when you cry because tear ducts from the eyes drain through the nose. When you smell delicious food, your stomach starts to secrete digestive acids before you even start eating. When you become dehydrated, you crave fluids. Day in and day out, there is virtually no limit to what a body does outside of conscious perception.

The intricate connection of one body system to another is true of every life form. But the human being is endowed with an organ more complicated than any other creature's on earth: the brain. While the body may seem to function autonomously, you can be sure that the brain continuously monitors, evaluates, and reacts to the internal processes of every other organ. In the healthy human body, nothing happens that the brain doesn't know about. And much of it happens outside of conscious awareness.

The brain is constantly learning about the state of the body. Sometimes it gets messages directly though nerve cells that turn on with a stimulus to cause conscious perception. For example, sticking yourself with a thorn will activate the pain receptors in your finger to send a message to your brain. In addition to birthing an increasing consciousness of your problem, that very same brain will send a message down to your arm, hand, and finger, instructing the muscles to launch a full-scale retreat from the rose stem. As an additional bonus, through a much different nerve pathway, your cerebral cortex launches a loud "Ouch!"

from your voice box before you even have a chance to think about it. These pathways to and from the brain happen in millionths of a second, and occur millions of times an hour. They inform the body about everything from the location of the lumps on your mattress to how low your husband turned the thermostat when you left the room.

The brain also finds out about what's happening below the cranium through another means altogether: hormones. When most of us hear "hormones" we think of psychotic body builders, PMS, or the raging hormones of adolescence. But hormones are more than chemicals that overtake people during sex-linked events. Technically, hormones are any material that travels in the blood from one organ to another with the purpose of changing that second organ's action. Insulin is a good example of a hormone. It gets produced in the pancreas, pours into the bloodstream after a meal, and acts on the "end organ" (the liver, muscle, and fat cells) to regulate sugar levels. Besides insulin, the body produces dozens of hormones, from thyroid (produced in a gland in the neck), which regulates metabolism, to calcitonin (produced near the thyroid), which helps strengthen bones. Each hormone acts like a microscopic messenger. When it arrives at its destination, it triggers a flood of chemical interactions that affect the rest of the body. Your body is awash in hormones, and they influence your life in remarkable ways.

Until recently, traditional medical science has paid scant attention to the effects of hormones on human behavior. Most psychopharmacologists recognize that brain chemicals such as serotonin or dopamine affect behavior. But these are chemicals that are synthesized and transported between nerve cells in the brain; as such, they are not hormones. In the last decade, brain science researchers have launched new investigations into how hormones play a critical role in thought processes. Melatonin, a hormone synthesized in the pineal gland, can regulate seasonal mood dips and correct insomnia; thyroid hormone can augment the uplifting effects of antidepressant medication; testosterone, produced in the sex organs of men and women, can increase energy levels; oxytocin, from the pituitary gland in the brain, can stimulate feelings of calm. Even some medications, such as Ketoconazole, invented to treat fungal infections, have been shown to affect the production of cortisol in the body and help elevate mood.

Today, in laboratories around the world, researchers probe the workings of the brain, looking for scientific explanations for the differences between men and women. The discoveries they have made so far do not reveal, as pop psychologists suggest, that men and women are from different planets. But the studies do prove what Sigmund Freud posited more than a century ago: Biology is destiny. And hormones drive that destiny.

In the second trimester of a woman's pregnancy, her developing baby sends out a code in its DNA that signals a barrage of hormones that mold that baby's brain and body. If the mother reads the code as "boy," by recognizing the XY chromosome, her body makes sure that fetus is flooded in testosterone. If the baby's DNA has an XX, the mother's body will decode that as "girl," and female hormones will deluge the womb. If my wife is more attuned to people's feelings and I am more engaged by a Victoria's Secret commercial, it is in large part due to the hormones we swam in between the third and sixth months after conception.

Exposure to these prenatal hormones affects behavior in two major ways. It changes physical structures of the body, and it changes the brain's response to other hormones that appear later in life. For instance, the part of the cerebral cortex that involves communication between lobes of the brain—the corpus callosum—is more developed in women than men; the anger center, the amygdala, is larger in men. Because female brains contain more oxytocin than men's brains, the bonding effects of this hormone draw women toward close connections with others. Men have lower oxytocin levels, but in contrast to women, they have up to twenty times more testosterone—the hormone responsible for aggression and sex drive. These chemical messengers, and dozens like them, act on the brain, impacting nearly all human activities.

Hormones surge though the body, yes, but the body's receptivity to hormones also develops during fetal stages. When puberty arrives, you can flood a young man with estrogen but he'll never grow breasts as a woman does. Women bodybuilders who use male steroids do get courser features, but they never lose all of their female attributes. That is because each end organ of a hormone must have receptors that stand ready to act once an expected hormone arrives. In women, there are many receptors that prepare for estrogen and progesterone throughout the

Day 1 Day 2 Day 3 Day 4 Day 5 Day 6 Day 7

body. In men, testosterone and vasopressin receptors await the arrival of their trigger hormones. It is only when the right hormone meets the right receptor that chemical changes begin to happen within the brain and body.

When it comes to women's physical state, we know a tremendous amount about the day-to-day changes that happen because of hormones' influences. Much of my medical school training in ob-gyn centered on the standard charts that show how the follicles in the ovaries change with increasing levels of estrogen, how progesterone increases the growth of endometrial cells, and finally how the dropoff in the levels of both of these hormones cause changes in bodily fluids, breast tissue density, and uterine lining. Indeed, by examining the body's signs, a physician can tell where a woman is in her menstrual cycle to within one day.

Now, twenty years after sitting for my first anatomy class, science has begun to apply that same rigor to figuring out what is happening inside a woman's brain during the menstrual cycle. And the results are stunning. In *28 Days*, Gabrielle Lichterman dives deeply into the scientific data that link hormonal changes in your body to behavior changes in your brain. Most women have predictable hormonal cycles during their reproductive years. The hormones estrogen, testosterone, and progesterone wash over brain cycles in a regular pattern. As they alternatively invade and retreat from your brain cells, these hormones stir up a predictable array of emotions, perceptions, and yearnings. Reproductive urges that overtake a woman during the first days of her cycle may color her perception of the ideal man. If she doesn't pay attention to the role that testosterone is playing in her bloodstream, she may find some stranger moving in with her weeks later—and she's stuck for months, or years, to come. Alternatively, a married woman may feel increasing animosity toward her husband in the last weeks of her cycle. As the progesterone levels rise, the decline in her verbal skills and energy level affect her feelings of competence. If a husband isn't sensitive to these changes in her, his attempts to "fix" the problem may be misinterpreted by his mate as not caring about her. These are the very conflicts that bring people to my office in search of marriage counseling. And these are the very things that can be avoided with knowledge of a woman's internal rhythm.

As you read the pages of *28 Days*, consider each of these hormones as you would characters in your life that enter and exit your home on a 28-day schedule. On the days that Aunt Edna and Uncle Phil come over, you can predict that things will drag on; when cousin Ruth stops by, you know you'll really have fun. But beware when Ruth and Edna are together, because the conversation can really get heated. So it is with the hormones that enter and exit your brain. Knowing what chemical messenger is knocking on your door each day will help you prepare for what's to come, and make the right choices for your day. This book introduces you to each of the characters and helps you to understand what they are, how they work, and how their presence, or absence, will affect you. To expand on Freud's insights: Knowing your biology can and will help you shape your destiny.

Day 1　Day 2　Day 3　Day 4　Day 5　Day 6　Day 7

So start now by learning about yourself. *28 Days* combines the wisdom of the ages with the cutting-edge science of the twenty-first century. In the pages that follow, you will explore the wonders of the female body. You will unravel mysteries of the mind. You will develop the tools to maximize your potential. Use these tools today, but don't stop there. Like the wonderful human form that inspired its creation, *28 Days* is for life.

Scott Haltzman, M.D.
Clinical Assistant Professor of
Psychiatry and Human Behavior
Brown University, Providence, Rhode Island

Introduction
You Are What You Secrete

Estrogen, testosterone, progesterone—a woman's "big three" hormones.[1] They've been around since, well, women have existed really. But with the massive amount of research being done about them lately, you'd think they were as new an addition to the female body as navel piercing.

Most of the hormone research you've heard about probably has to do with menopause, perimenopause, postmenopause, and hormone replacement therapy—basically, all having to do with a woman who's already *losing* her hormones.

But what about a gal like you—who's menstruating and still producing plenty of estrogen, testosterone, and progesterone? Aren't researchers interested in knowing how hormones affect *your* mind and body?

Yes, they are. In fact, there are hundreds of recent studies about how these three hormones affect healthy, menstruating women. And what the studies reveal is that estrogen, testosterone, and progesterone have powerful effects on just about every aspect of your life—your mood, memory, verbal ability, concentration, ability to learn new facts, the kind of guy you're attracted to, your libido, the intensity and ease of orgasms, how you spend money, and your energy level. And that's just the short list!

Day 1   Day 2   Day 3   Day 4   Day 5   Day 6   Day 7

But the biggest revelation of all? The way your hormone levels combine has a different effect on you each day of your menstrual cycle. This means that on some days, your hormones will make you feel as outgoing and upbeat as Kelly Ripa and other days they'll make you feel more reclusive than Ted Kaczynski. On some days, your hormones will make you speak as flawlessly as a newscaster and on other days they'll make words like "specificity" and "apoplectic" give your tongue a cramp. On some days, your hormones will make you attracted to masculine-looking guys with a strong jaw and sexy stubble and on other days they'll make you prefer more feminine-looking guys who couldn't grow a beard after a Rogaine facial.

How can hormones have such a profound effect on so much in your life? Because hormones are potent molecules. In fact, sometimes all it takes is a mere *billionth* of a gram to have an effect. And throughout your menstrual cycle, your hormones are either rising or falling, which means their potent effects change every single day.

Now, this doesn't mean that your whole personality and everything you do is entirely controlled by your hormones. They're more like a major influence. Okay, a *really* major influence. So having a clearer understanding of how they're affecting you on a day-to-day basis can actually give you *more* control over your life.

How so? Well, there are some hormonal effects you can acknowledge and decide to follow if you want to (such as buying impulse items on Day 1 or cheating on your boyfriend on Day 14). There are other hormonal effects you can't change, but you can work around (such as writing down facts you need to remember on Day 28, when your memory is low, or reminding yourself to show some excitement when your boyfriend asks you to marry him on Day 22, when you're at your most subdued). Still other hormonal effects can help you determine the best days to schedule events (for instance, you'll enjoy your vacation more if you take it during Days 4 to 13, when your mood is most upbeat and open to new experiences, and you'll be more successful asking for a raise on Day 10, when high confidence and sharp brain skills combine to have you making the best possible case to your boss).

While estrogen, testosterone, and progesterone produce predictable effects in menstruating women, they don't produce cookie-cutter results. Rather, these hormones determine where you are within the spectrum of your own personality. For instance, one woman's throwing caution to the wind on Day 11 may mean slapping on a pair of gold lamé go-go boots and dancing on the bar at Hogs & Heifers. For another woman, it may mean wearing a V-neck. For one woman, being in the height of her verbal, memory, and cognitive cycles on Day 13 may mean she makes a breakthrough in neuroscience. For another woman, it may mean she writes a kick-ass term paper on Bob Dylan. It's all relative.

Is it antifeminist to say a woman isn't as smart or her memory isn't as good on certain days? Well, it's not as if women gain and lose 100 IQ points in the course of a cycle. They simply range between ordinary brain skills, when estrogen and testosterone are low, and extraordinary brain skills, when estrogen and testosterone are high.

What's more, regardless of the day in their menstrual cycle, women tend to outperform guys in most areas. Oh sure, men may often have the edge on gals when it comes to math, mazes, and spatial relationships.[2] But women pretty much outshine men at everything else. In fact, women generally test 3 percent higher on intelligence tests.[3] Plus, they have more gray matter in their brain (which is where you do your computational work and communicating), have better communication between the left and right hemispheres of their brain, have superior verbal abilities, grasp languages more easily, and have sharper memories.[4] There's lots more stuff gals also do better than guys, but why rub it in?[5]

Is it politically incorrect to say women are influenced by their hormones? Well, it's not just women who are influenced by hormones. Men have estrogen, progesterone and testosterone, too, and they're just as influenced by them.[6] Besides, while women go through a monthly cycle of highs and lows, men experience a cycle of highs and lows every single day.[7] So if you want to talk about mood swings . . .

If hormones have such a powerful effect over so much of your daily life, how come you don't know about them yet? Well, to give the doctors and researchers credit, they have constantly provided new information, but the information has been scattered in hundreds of different places.

28 Days is the first book to compile these hundreds of hormone studies into one handy day-by-day guide that you can follow along with your cycle. It will help you plan your day, week, and month as never before.

Gabrielle Lichterman
Day 11, New York City
Book Web site: *www.28Days-thebook.com*
Author e-mail: Gabrielle@28Days-thebook.com

How to Use This Book

Do you have to start on Day 1?

You can start reading *28 Days* any day of your menstrual cycle. Simply turn to whatever day you're on in your cycle and read that chapter right now!

How can you tell what day you're on?

Count how many days it's been since the first day of your last period. That's what day you're on today!

Do you have a "perfect" 28-day menstrual cycle?

Then read one chapter each day of your cycle. Day 1 is the first day of your period.

Do you take hormone contraceptives that suppress ovulation—such as the pill, the mini pill, Ortho Evra patch, NuvaRing, Lunelle, Depo-Provera, or Seasonale?

If you take 28-day hormone contraceptives, then read one chapter each day of your cycle. Day 1 is the first day of your period—*not* the first day your contraceptive's hormones begin.

Day 1   Day 2   Day 3   Day 4   Day 5   Day 6   Day 7

If you take a 91-day hormone contraceptive (such as Seasonale), read one chapter from Day 1 to Day 5. Day 1 is the first day of your period—*not* the first day your contraceptive's hormones begin. Then when your hormones kick in on Day 6, read each chapter for four days till Day 28. This will match up with your 91-day menstrual cycle.

Is your cycle longer or shorter than 28 days? Does the length of your cycle vary from month to month?
28 Days works for any length menstrual cycle. Even cycles that change from month to month.

Here's how to follow the chapters so *28 Days* fits your personal cycle:

Starting on Day 1: Read one chapter a day until you ovulate. (How to know when you ovulate is coming up in a sec.)

On the day you ovulate: Read Day 14. If you ovulate before you reach the 14th day of your cycle, jump ahead to Day 14. If you haven't ovulated by the 14th day of your cycle, reread Day 13 till you ovulate. Whatever day you end up ovulating is *your* Day 14.

Days 15 to 28: Read one chapter a day for the rest of your cycle. The second half of a woman's cycle is usually a consistent 14 days, so you'll match up no matter how long your cycle is!

Day 8 Day 9 Day 10 Day 11 Day 12 Day 13 Day 14

How can you tell when you're ovulating?

Look for one or more of these telltale signs:

- Your vaginal fluid is thinner and slicker, like egg white
- You feel a dull cramp near your ovary
- Your libido suddenly increases

Or use these two easy methods for tracking ovulation:

- To find out when it's one day *before* ovulation: Use a "saliva ovulation tester," a reusable lipstick-shaped mini-microscope that determines when you're about to ovulate by measuring the amount of salt in your saliva. When estrogen peaks, so does the salt in your saliva. And that indicates that it's one day before ovulation. You can purchase a reusable saliva ovulation tester in drugstores or online for $20 to $60.
- To find out when it's one day *after* ovulation: Take your "basal temperature" every day. That's your body temperature right after waking but before getting out of bed. On the day after you ovulate, your basal temperature rises .5 to one degree Fahrenheit. For the most accurate results, use a "basal thermometer," an ultrasensitive thermometer that tracks your body's subtlest temperature shifts. You can purchase a basal thermometer at drugstores or online for about $6 to $20.

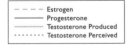

Day 1 Day 2 Day 3 Day 4 Day 5 Day 6 Day 7

Follow your cycle with the *28 Days* Hormone Chart!
Your natural estrogen, testosterone, and progesterone levels rise and fall throughout your menstrual cycle. This chart makes it easy to follow these ups and downs every day.

When looking at testosterone levels, pay closer attention to the "testosterone perceived" line. This shows you how much your body *feels* testosterone, as opposed to how much your body is producing. Because there isn't as much research available on exact levels of perceived testosterone, this line is an estimate based on estrogen and progesterone's known impact on perceived testosterone.

Taking hormone contraceptives? Then your hormone peaks likely won't be as high and your valleys as low as those with natural hormones.

28 Days Hormone Chart

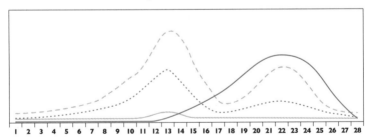

– – –	Estrogen
———	Progesterone
———	Testosterone Produced
·········	Testosterone Perceived

Your Period's Here— And It's Brought Friends!

Day 1

Mood

TV commercials no longer make you cry. Your mood ring has stopped changing color every six minutes. And your mate's taken the padlock off the knife drawer. All this can mean just one thing—PMS is officially over!

Within hours of getting your period, the dark cloud that's been hanging over your head this past week evaporates quicker than a plate of fat-free brownies at a Weight Watchers convention. Gone are the depression and crying jags, and you're no longer flying off the handle at little things you'd overlook the rest of the month, like your guy breathing.

Why the sudden change, Miss Flipside? After plummeting for the past few days, estrogen finally begins to rise today.[1] And if a woman's happiness is caused by one thing, it's—okay, it's diamonds. But if it's caused by *two* things, it's diamonds and rising estrogen.

That's because once estrogen starts to increase, it puts the brakes on the estrogen withdrawal that's been causing PMS.[2] Think of it as a kind of hair of the dog. Just like that morning swig after a night of heavy drinking, a little estrogen goes a long way toward making a hormone hangover disappear.

But curing PMS isn't the only reason estrogen deserves the revered position as girl's second best friend. When on the rise, this hormone also revs up the positive feelings that are the trademarks of Days 1 to 13, such as optimism, extroversion, and a desire to have the kind of fun that leaves you wondering where you left your panties and when you got that tattoo.[3]

As if that wasn't enough, when estrogen rises, it also boosts your level of testosterone.[4] And when this hormone increases, it pumps up the self-assured feelings that are the other trademarks of Days 1 to 13, such as assertiveness, competitiveness, and the kind of confidence that has you pretty sure you can snag the corner office by lunch and the phone number of that cute guy on the fifth floor by sundown.

Positive feelings? Self-assuredness? Putting the kibosh on PMS? Is there nothing estrogen and testosterone can't do?

Well, don't break out the victory champagne just yet. These happiness-inducing hormones may be taking the elevator to the top, but they're still only at the first floor. Plus, you're putting up with lots today—cramps, tummy aches, backaches, headaches, joint aches, and the nagging feeling that you'll never live a day without pain again.

Rest assured, by Day 3, when estrogen and testosterone reach even higher levels, you'll be looking at the

empty Motrin bottles scattered around you like shell cas-
ings after a battle, wondering what all the fuss was about.

Until then, you're happiest curling up with some
empty calories and the remote. And tell the boy-toy to be
on standby for a Motrin run.

What's on TV?

From Day 1 to Day 5, you prefer sitcoms, funny movies, or any other kind of show that makes you laugh.
Low on your to-watch list: dramas and tear jerkers,
the news, or anything else too serious. Research
shows women use humorous TV programs to distract themselves from the aches and pains of menstruation.[5] But networks know the real truth: We
can just never get enough *Friends* repeats.

Mind

Two things you should know: The first is that the higher
estrogen and testosterone go, the better your brain function. The second is that, even though they're both on the
rise today, estrogen and testosterone are starting out at
rock bottom, which means your brain function is at rock-
bottom, too. Some good news? Your creative right brain is
peaking, which makes you way more inventive at covering
up any cognitive slipups that come with low hormones.

Thinking

You've got the attention span of an MTV target audience member. You're reading the microwave popcorn directions ten times before you finally get them. And you're standing in the frozen foods aisle for what seems like twenty minutes trying to decide which brand of waffles to buy.[6] Having a Jessica Simpson kinda day? No doubt. But don't worry—as estrogen and testosterone rise, your focus increases, fuzzy thinking disappears, and you make decisions in nanoseconds.[7] Till then, take solace in the fact that no matter how brain-dead you feel today, your mind is still functioning better than most men on their best days.[8]

Memory

Since when did trying to find your keys turn into a more daunting hunt than the search for WMDs? Since estrogen and testosterone bottomed out yesterday and today—that's when. Oh, you could try to write down things you need to remember or type them in to your Blackberry. But what's the use when you forget to look at them? Better off to simply plead a premature senior moment and cut yourself some slack.

Verbal

Ah, high estrogen days—a time when SAT words came spilling from your mouth as easily as prescription pills out of Courtney Love's handbag. And now? You're lucky you can spit out "Motrin run" without giving your tongue a cramp. Don't worry, though, not many people will notice your verbal tie-up since low estrogen has you feeling quiet and less into chatting anyway.[9]

The side of your brain highlighted today?

Right brain: Sure, from the outside it looks as if you're so exhausted you can barely stir a packet of Splenda into your decaf cappuccino. (To be fair, the foam is rather thick.) But on the inside, your mind is a whirling hamster wheel of creativity! That's because since Day 20, your hormones have handed the controls over to your right brain—the free-spirited Phoebe to your color-inside-the-lines, left-brain Monica. During this phase brainstorming is a breeze, problem solving is a snap, and coming up with new ideas is as easy as reaching your credit card limit.

During your right brain phase, your thoughts turn inward and you're reflecting on the many issues in your life. One minute you may be questioning if you're on the right career path. The next minute, you're wondering if chartreuse is really your color.

You're also better at writing, which definitely makes blog ranting so much easier. And you're more comfortable working in messy piles than in organized space. So when your cubicle mate asks why you don't straighten up the place, you can tell him it's because of your right brain. (Or to shove it. Totally your call.)

Romance

If you're in a relationship . . .

Tell your sweetie it's safe for him to come back home. After narrowly escaping another PMS, he'll probably think it's a trap and need convincing. But truth is, a few hours after getting your period, you'll be feeling lovey-dovey once again.

Why the change of heart? Well, you know those cramps you've been having? They're caused by the hormone oxytocin. And it turns out that, in addition to causing nerve-crunching uterine pain, this chemical also increases how bonded you feel to your honey.

Who'da thunk it—a woman's most hated hormone is also a veritable Cupid! Perhaps it's some sort of karmic refund for all the hurting and tears. Or maybe it's evolution's way of coaxing your guy back into the house to take another shot at fertilization later on in the month. Whatever the reason, every time you feel a cramp down below, consider it an arrow shot directly from Cupid's bow bringing you closer to your mate.

If you're single . . .

Men who try to pick you up today can thank oxytocin if they succeed. Besides causing uterine cramps during menstruation, this hormone also boosts your feelings of trust. [10] The result? You're more likely to buy whatever dubious line a guy comes up with. For example, when he says he's a billionaire, or that the ring tan on his left hand is just a spot the spray-on missed.

Sex

Cramps. Premenstrual acne that hasn't cleared up yet. Bloat that makes every pair of pants you try on the one you hate more. Everyone who thinks this has low libido written all over it, raise your hand.

Not so fast, Day 1 Girl. Turns out, despite pain, zits, and a body as swollen as a Hollywood starlet's lips, your libido is turned up high today. Give in to your carnal cravings with sex or masturbation and you'll also discover that orgasms are not only easy to reach, but are top-dollar toe curlers.

What's fueling this libidinous lust-for-all? Congestion in your uterus as well as today's rise in estrogen and testosterone. Even though these two hormones increase only a tiny amount, it's enough to rev up your sex drive and make going for an orgasm totally worth being late to your Pilates class.

How so? For starters, testosterone is giving you that gotta-have-it-or-die-trying feeling. It's also filling your head with naughty thoughts when you should be paying attention to other, more important things, such as a client at a business meeting or a smoke alarm alerting you to a kitchen fire.[11] Testosterone also heightens the sensation in your nipples and clitoris, helps you reach climax faster, and it gives your orgasms their intensity.[12]

If testosterone does all that, what's left for estrogen to do? A small, but oh-so-important part: lubrication.[13] The female equivalent of a male erection, lubrication is a barometer of how turned on you are. And so just like sex can't happen with a Mr. Softee, without lubrication, you may as well be trying to bowl a strike in the Sahara.

Think it's ironic that a woman's sex drive is so high when many women prefer to sit it out on the sidelines till menstruation is over? Well, evolution may have had a hand in this oddly timed libido boost. It turns out there are a few health advantages to orgasming during your period. It can relieve menstrual cramps by pushing out the menstrual fluid and relieving tension in your uterine muscles.[14] It's been shown to reduce your risk of developing endometriosis.[15] As if that's not enough, it increases feel-good brain chemicals such as serotonin, dopamine, and endorphins, which improve mood and decrease pain.[16]

Wish period sex wasn't so messy?

Want to take advantage of your high libido and get all the health benefits from orgasming during your period—but don't want to deal with the "ick factor" or sacrifice your favorite designer sheets in the process? There's a simple solution: Use the Instead Softcup, the latest alternative to pads and tampons. Shaped like a diaphragm, the Instead Softcup fits over your cervix to neatly collect flowing blood, making it perfect for mess-free sex. And talk about discreet—your guy won't even notice you have one in! The Instead Softcup is sold at most major drugstores and online at *www.softcup.com*.

Money

Rising testosterone makes you impulsive.[17] Rising estrogen pumps up your optimism, which makes you feel as though you've got money to burn. Together, this freewheeling combo has you spending dough like you were born a Hilton, and has you heading straight for the definitely-not-a-necessity items—such as a diamond-studded tiara or a toaster that toasts Hello Kitty's face on every slice.

But splurge-loving estrogen and testosterone aren't limiting themselves to just big-ticket purchases. They're also pushing you to fill your basket with little items you had no plans to buy but which seem oddly irresistible today, such as candy, magazines, miniflashlights, glow-in-the-dark rulers—basically anything placed next to a cash register. Don't want to break the bank? Hide the credit cards somewhere you're not likely to go today, like the vegetable crisper.

Career

Work? Shmerk! Curling up in your chair and a half watching *Blind Date* reruns seems so much more tempting.

However, if you do end up being one of the nearly three out of four menstruating women who manage to drag their tired, achy selves in to office today, you're bringing lots to the table.[18] Like what? How about amazing, out-of-the-box ideas! With your creative right brain surging, you're the go-to gal for anyone who needs a new plan, fresh perspective, or solution so imaginative it makes the person who thought up the phrase "wardrobe malfunction" seem uninspired.

Have something to say, such as proposing a project or giving a presentation? Schedule it for Days 6 to 10 when higher levels of estrogen and testosterone have you running verbal circles around the competition. Can't put it off until then? Then put it in writing. Low estrogen may have you tongue-tied, but your right brain is making you utterly eloquent on paper. So jot down all those brilliant ideas you're coming up with. There's a good chance you won't remember them tomorrow (or in an hour), since the same low estrogen and testosterone that are giving you so many great ideas are also making your memory hit the lowest point of its cycle.

Energy

Estrogen and testosterone are hormones that you can usually count on to inject you with vitality and stamina. But with both so low today, even after they begin to rise they won't be enough to scrape you off the bed sheets. As a result, you'll likely spend the day feeling lethargic, listless, and longing to take a nap.

To be fair, this lack of get-up-and-go isn't all low estrogen and testosterone's fault. The bleeding from menstruation is also contributing to your exhaustion because it's depleting you of iron—a mineral in red blood cells that gives you energy. Think that menstrual blood is "extra" so it doesn't count? Not so. Your body feels the deenergizing effects of losing blood whether it's from menstruation or a cut while shaving.[19] Well, a really big cut, anyway.

Looking for some extra pep during the day? Then skip the java joint. Caffeine may give you a temporary lift, but it'll burn up whatever iron you've got left, making you even more exhausted once the caffeine buzz wears off.[20] Better to pop an iron supplement or load up on iron-rich foods, such as meat, eggs, dark vegetables, and iron-enriched cereal. (Yes, Lucky Charms counts!)

Diet

You're in the mood for waffles, chocolate chip cookies, cheeseburgers, fries, malted milkshakes, and other familiar comfort foods while estrogen and testosterone are low.[21]

The good news is you don't have to feel guilty about eating all those yummy fats, carbs, salts, and sugars. Okay, well not *too* guilty. Now that progesterone's gone, you're eating 12 percent less than you have in the last two weeks[22] and you're no longer hit with hunger pangs after just three to four hours.[23] Plus, while it may not feel like it, you're not craving off-limit treats with the same gotta-eat-it-or-I'll-die way you did from Days 14 to 28.[24] Then why are you still feeling a gravitational pull toward these nutritional no-nos? Newsflash: Junk food is addictive![25] But without progesterone bullying you into the bakery aisle, you have a better chance at kicking the high-cal habit from today till Day 13.

Health

Even though estrogen and testosterone rise just a smidge today, it's enough to have a powerful effect on many aspects of your health:

- With progesterone gone and estrogen rising, your breasts are less tender and the bloating and constipation you experienced during the second half of your cycle ends.[26]
- Your immune system takes a hit today through Day 5: You're 30 percent more susceptible to allergic reactions than on Day 13. There's also a higher probability of acne, bacterial infection, hives, herpes sores, irritable bowel syndrome flare-ups, tonsillitis, and ulcer attacks. It's not all bad news, though—you're warding off colds and flus better.[27]
- If you're a smoker who wants to quit, you'll be more successful if you kick the habit today through Day 13. That's because rising estrogen makes nicotine withdrawal less severe than Days 14 to 28.[28]
- Brush and floss your teeth more often from today until Day 5. During menstruation, the glucose content of your saliva increases three- to ninefold. This increases bacteria in your mouth that cause gum infection and tooth decay.[29]
- Asthma alert: 75 percent of asthma attacks occur either during or shortly before menstruation.[30]
- Migraine alert: Today through Day 3 are high-risk days for menstrual migraine.[31] So avoid migraine triggers, such as caffeine, citrus fruits, salt, and food preservatives.[32]

Look out!

Low estrogen and testosterone are making your coordination poor[33] and reaction time slow.[34] So you might want to skip the water ballet practice in your Endless pool, which could prove disastrous without high estrogen and testosterone to keep you balanced. Ditto for square dancing, which, it's been said, requires the coordination of a stunt pilot.

But there's a silver lining: When estrogen gets as low as it is today, your ability to judge distances and direction reaches its month-long high.[35] Sooo, while you may be less able to reduce someone to tears with a cleverly worded insult on a low estrogen day, you will be able to nail them square in the temple with a Jimmy Choo sling-back at forty paces with alarming accuracy.

Ouchers!

When estrogen is low, it lowers your level of endorphins—a brain neurotransmitter that lessens your sensitivity to pain. And today your estrogen is pretty darned low, making you feel extra sensitive to aches, pains, and even the softest touches.[36] Silk jammies feel like they're made out of steel wool. Your pillow feel as if someone jammed igneous rocks into it while you were sleeping. And high heels are certainly some kind of karmic punishment for wearing pleather in a past life.

PMS prevention starts on Day 1

Studies show taking a multivitamin every day of the month can dramatically reduce the symptoms of PMS.[37]

Prevent painful cramps

Take ibuprofen (like Advil or Motrin) before cramps even begin. This will decrease the production of prostaglandins—hormonelike substances that cause the inflammation and pain of menstrual cramps. The result? Your cramps will be milder or you may prevent them altogether![38]

Let the Positive Spin Begin

Mood

The sun burns a little brighter. Birds sing a little sweeter. And tofu burgers taste more like the real thing. Don't worry, no one's slipped a Prozac into your bubble tea. It's just rising estrogen and testosterone slipping a pair of rose-colored Ray-Bans on you that make you see the world as a beautiful place to be. Bad news for goth girls and broody Sofia Coppola. Good news if you like living in a place where people seem nicer and the traffic less congested, and being forced to watch thirty-five minutes of premovie commercials feels a little less like cruel and unusual punishment.

But make no mistake—you're not turning you into a total Teflon-coated Stepford wife, with all of life's annoyances instantly bouncing off your peppy exterior. You'll still get angry if, say, someone dents your car or (gosh forbid) finishes off the Marshmallow Fluff. But rising estrogen and testosterone will help you get over it a lot more easily and return you quickly to your regularly scheduled joy.

There's just one thing you should be wary of while

enjoying this positive state of mind: You're tempted to over-look obvious dangers. Such as? Such as that surly waiters would never give you a sneezer. (Not true, keep an eye out for suspicious globules.) And that the guy you met through Prison PenPals seems too sweet to be guilty of double mur-der. (It's best to wait for the DNA results to come in before inviting him over for a post-release brunch.)

With the world looking so wonderful now and your hormones giving you a slight energy boost, like a game of double dutch jump rope, you're probably thinking about the right place to jump in. Maybe go to the club and dance the night away in a sea of nameless faces and (with any luck) rock-hard abs. Head to a sultry candlelit bôite with velvet banquettes, upon which you'll daringly get to sec-ond base with your honey beside other pretzel-twisted canoodling couples. Or opt for coffee for one at the chic new café, which may be a bit overlit but is perfect for showing off your killer new lipstick.

But these are still just thoughts. Your energy may be on the rise but it's still just getting off the ground floor. Coupled with leftover aches and pains, you're happier at home munching on some Jiffy Pop and watching *South Park* rather than painting the town MAC Red.

Mind

Your brain skills sharpen as estrogen and testosterone rise. However, these two hormones are increasing just a smidge today, so the improvement is, well, a tad subtle.

Thinking

A plate of Krispy Kremes. A tanned hard-body who walks by your cubicle. A biscotti crumb lodged between your *A* and *S* keys. It seems that focus is so hard to keep when such important things like these pop up.

Learning something new today, say, step aerobics or the relative use of string theory in medicine? You may feel as though you don't get it on the first try and have to ask for instructions twice. Okay, three times. All right, you'll want to ask at least five times, but you'll give up around six and resolve to figure it out at home after *The Daily Show*.

It's easier to pull on control-top pantyhose than it is to make decisions since you're still a tad waffley on what you really want. So if you've got a big choice to make—whether to buy a new car, for example—before you sign on the dotted line, consider holding off till Day 6. That's when estrogen and testosterone rise enough to make decision-making so much easier. And it gives the car salesman a few days to sweat it out and come up with a better offer.

Memory

Okay, so you found the keys in the freezer. Now if only you can remember where you left your dignity after you called your date by the wrong name.

Verbal

Friends don't have to worry about you hogging the conversation since you're on the quiet side today. However, by Day 4, you'll be a regular chatty Kathy Griffin again.

So they should get all that boring crap about themselves in while they still can.

The side of your brain highlighted today?

Right brain: You can use right brain creativity to help solve practically any problem. Your boss prowling the corridors demanding a cost-cutting idea from every employee? You hit him with your idea to substitute pricey Post-Its with recycled paper and chewing gum. Your next-door neighbor insists on mowing his lawn at 5:00 A.M.? You replace his grass with Astro Turf in the middle of the night.

Your writing skills are also sharper during your right brain phase. So if creative genius didn't fix your problems, perhaps aiming your pen at it will. For instance, maybe scribble down your money-saving proposal on one of your ingenious Gum-Its and stick it on your boss's Prada leather briefcase. Or slip a note in your inconsiderate neighbor's mailbox and dare to get all UPPERCASE on him.

With your right brain making you introspective, you'll probably feel like mulling over a few important issues in your life. Whether to eat or skip the jelly-filled doughnut, however, is not one of these issues.

Romance

If you're in a relationship . . .

Sure, he uses your apricot face scrub to clean the grease off his tools. And his idea of a fancy dinner is a bucket of KFC with cloth napkins. But with your penchant for emphasizing the positives during rising estrogen days, you're focusing on his good side and all that he does to make you happy—for instance, the way he wears the pink polo shirt you gave him, no matter how wussy it makes him feel, and how he totally caves at the first sign of a tear.

Cherish this rosy-hued feeling, but don't let your guy think of it as an official pardon. Continue to work on important issues. Otherwise, when Day 23 rolls around and the reality of his shortcomings comes into tight focus once again, you may be tempted to kick him and his well-scrubbed tools out the door.

If you're single . . .

You're feeling hopeful about finding a partner—it's not matter of "if" but "when." In anticipation of this month's search for Mr. Right, you're making a mental wish list of what you want in a soul mate—"sk8tr" boy versus corporate cutie, young gun versus older sophisticate, Luke Wilson versus Owen Wilson. Do the future you a favor and put your list in writing. Then laminate it and carry it around wherever you go. Don't have pockets? Then tattoo the list somewhere on your body. It's *that* important. And you'll see why on Days 13, 14, and 15, when your hormones propel you, like a Ping-Pong ball out of a Bangkok bar girl's yoo-hoo, toward guys you wouldn't accept a free drink from the rest of the month.

Sex

If you don't mind a little cleanup, or if you plan to use your helpful Instead Softcup to keep things tidy, you'll be leaving a trail of crunchy Cheetos from the TV to the bedroom for your guy to follow.

Taking matters into your own hands? Then holy carpal tunnel, Batgirl, you may need to ice your wrist after today! That's because rising testosterone is revving up your libido, increasing the sensitivity in your nipples and clitoris, and, thankfully, interrupting boring tasks with many steamy daydreams. Once you give in to testosterone-driven desire, you'll find that orgasms are easy to reach and forceful enough to blow your nipple rings right off.

Want to supersize your sex drive?

Indulge in your favorite alcoholic drink! Turns out, liquor does indeed make gals want to hop into bed, just as generations of horny frat boys hoped. But it's not for the reason they think. Dudes do not, repeat, do not get more attractive the more a woman drinks. Beer goggles is a phenomenon that occurs only in men.[1] So what makes alcohol work its libido-boosting magic in women? Alcohol raises your testosterone level, which in turn, increases your sex drive.[2] So while you get hornier, he doesn't get hunkier. He's gotta have the goods before the drinks are even poured.

Money

Got bills? Of course you do! They got you? Not a chance. With optimism rising, you're certain you can earn enough money (at least one day) to pay off everything. You may even feel so flush with cash that you can afford to give a few dollars to an animal shelter, local charity, or that coworker who's dealing her daughter's Girl Scout cookies out of her cubicle like a support-hosed drug pusher. (And who doesn't know at least one gal who's needed a Thin Mint intervention?)

You're also spending more on impulse items as testosterone rises. And with your brain not yet in its logical left brain phase, a little thing like price doesn't bother you. So the card's the limit on whatever catches your eye and makes you forget all about your low estrogen aches and pains and second-day cramps.

Career

No doubt your job has its flaws—the pay is weak, the cubicle is the size of a pad of sticky notes, and every year your Secret Santa gets you another freakin' Chia Pet. But rising estrogen and testosterone have you looking on the bright side: at least they fired your cubicle-mate with the pit stains the size of watermelons, you're stealing your weight in paper clips, and you can always regift that Chia Pet the next time an office birthday rolls around.

Now that it looks as though you won't be handing in that letter of resignation after all, it's time to start sucking up to the boss again. And what better way than to show off the talent your right brain's highlighting today—creative thinking. Use it to invent a brand-new filing system. Or dream up an innovative way to save your company millions that doesn't involve massive layoffs, outsourcing, or taking the cappuccino machine out of the lunchroom.

Once you've got your promotion-winning idea, put it in writing. Low estrogen is causing a few verbal blunders and your right brain makes you more persuasive on paper than in spoken word. Plus, it gives human resources something positive to put in your personnel file, which could come in handy should they ever find out about those paper clips.

Energy

You're feeling your first stirrings of pep from rising estrogen and testosterone. But this kick-start is deceiving. While you may wake up feeling as though you can run a long-distance marathon, your body will likely lose steam by the afternoon.

Instead of blowing today's teeny bit of energy by doing stuff that can be put off—such as, say, cleaning the fridge or answering calls from bill collectors—take it slow and steady. You'll be energized enough in the days ahead to throw out the moldy cottage cheese and, well, screw the bill collectors. Isn't that what you got caller ID for anyway?

Tonight your sleep will be deeper and more restful. You can thank rising estrogen for the extra ZZZs. It's increasing endorphins, which decreases the sensitivity to odors, sounds, and pains that have been keeping you awake this past week.

Diet

Doritos, Hostess snack cakes, Krispy Kremes, and other empty calorie comfort foods have less of a pull on you as estrogen and testosterone increase, making it easier to eat healthy. Okay, health*ier*.

However, even though these hormones are on the rise, they're still at relatively low levels. This means you're craving familiar dishes and are shying away from culinary risks, like an untried restaurant, exotic recipe, or your mate's meatloaf surprise.

Confidence Kicks In

Mood

You're standing a bit taller. Talking a little louder. Walking with a strut that lets everyone know you are all that. All because estrogen and testosterone continue to rise, and that's kicking your confidence up a notch. Of course, it also doesn't hurt that your premenstrual acne is clearing up and, since you're no longer retaining fluid like a water bottle on legs, you can fit into a pair of tight jeans again.

But confidence is giving you more than just a delicious-looking booty. (And it is delicious-looking.) It's also giving you the power to fight evil, cure alopecia, and have x-ray vision. Really? No. But till Day 13 it does give you a go-for-it attitude and the feeling that you won't be turned down no matter what you ask for. And that's just as good because it means you'll be creating opportunities and jumping on once-in-a-lifetime chances that come your way. Such as? Maybe pitching a new project to the company president when you spot him in the elevator. (Which would, of course, also involve a bonus and your own parking space.) Or persuading U2's road manager to take you on as a roadie. (It's not considered stalking if you're setting up guitars and schlepping amps.)

When it comes to socializing, you're on the fence. On one hand, rising estrogen and testosterone are making your mood brighter and giving you more energy. And you haven't spent the night carousing with friends in what seems like forever. On the other hand, while on the upswing, estrogen and testosterone are still at relatively low levels, so you're preferring places that are familiar and comfortable. And that makes staying in and ordering a pizza and a Pay Per View seem much more enticing. Why limit yourself to just one choice? Call up your buds and have them come over to your place. An added bonus: They may even bring dessert. Sweet!

Mind

Rising estrogen and testosterone continue to improve your brain skills. And just in time for you to want to show them off. Handy!

Thinking

You're learning new information easily and making decisions a tad faster. What's more, your ability to focus is better than it has been in days. So, if the office drama queen wants to distract you from your tasks with details of her latest faux-verdose, she's going to have to try a little harder. Your powers of concentration are so strong, you'll be tuning her out like a lecture on abstinence.

Memory

You're remembering more details today. Okay, so you may still be forgetting a couple of facts or names. But isn't that what personal assistants are for? Well, that and braving a hurricane to get you a mocha frappe.

Verbal

Hope you got those cell phone batteries charged while you had the chance. Quiet time is over and you're itching to get back in the gabbing game. But pace yourself. You're still experiencing a few verbal slipups. For example, you'll likely notice a few hesitations in your speech. Or you may say the wrong word, as in "I had the breast of intentions" when of course you meant "best," or "I would like a raise" when you really meant "I wish I had Bill Gates' kind of money so I could buy your company and fire your sorry-excuse-for-a-boss's ass."

The side of your brain highlighted today?

Right brain: Creative genius forever! Or at least till Day 6 when logic takes its place. So if you've got any inventions you want to get out before then, say, glitter hair dye or purses for pooches, get 'em in when imagination is still at its highest.

Introspection and intuition are also still strong. So if while you're mulling over an issue you get a hunch about a solution, go with it. It couldn't be any worse than what Miss Cleo had to offer.

Romance

If you're in a relationship . . .

Rising testosterone is building up the confidence you have in your relationship and in your choice of guys. No matter what anyone else says, he's your man and you'll defend him to the bitter end: He's not unemployed—he's devoting his life to working on his one-man show. He's not too broke to get a car—he's simply into saving the planet. He's not cheap—he's just saving for a really, really big ring. At least he'd better be.

If you're single...

You're feeling inspired to take action to find a special someone. However, after a third straight day of bleeding, you're not up for hitting the booty bar just yet. But with confidence in your appearance high, you are willing to swap pix on Match.com with a hard rock–lovin' accountant or exchange ironic poses on Nerve.com with an artsy intellectual who has a keen sense for fashionable eyewear.

Sex

You're throwing the sweats in the back of the closet, breaking out the pushup bra, and sending out the signals to your boy-toy that you're ready for love. Or at least lust. That's because rising testosterone is increasing your libido, making your nipples and clitoris more sensitive, and giving you easy-to-reach orgasms that are so ginormous you'll be making the neighbors jealous. And not just the ones next door, either.

Want to supersize your sex drive?

Brew a cup of green tea, down a Red Bull, slurp a Frappuccino at any one of the fifty-eight Starbucks that are within a mile of where you're sitting right now, or consume any other caffeinated beverage or snack. Research shows caffeine can give a mild boost to your estrogen level.[1] And the higher your estrogen goes, the more lust-loving testosterone rises, which charges up your libido!

Money

With don't-worry-about-a-little-thing-like-price testosterone on the rise, it feels as though you've got Oprah money to throw around. And don't-need-it-but-would-really-love-to-have-it estrogen is making luxury items—like an hour of Thai massage or, say, a Jacob watch with more ice than the Antarctic—seem especially tempting. Wanna keep some of that cash in your purse in case you need to eat later in the month? Then do not pass Gucci. Do not collect $200 worth of coordinating accessories.

Career

Is it you or is your job actually more enjoyable? It's you. Specifically your estrogen and testosterone, which are making you more confident about your work performance. And, really, why shouldn't you be? You're full of creative ideas. Your brain skills are getting sharper by the minute. And, if it came down to it, you're pretty sure you could take your supervisor in a mud-wrestling pit.

Now that you've realized what a valuable asset you are to the company, you may feel like storming into your boss's office to demand a raise and promotion. But before you do, consider this: Your verbal, cognitive, and memory skills really start to take off on Day 6. So try to put off your requests until then. That way, you can give an even more convincing argument for why you deserve the double-digit pay increase and juicier job title. (And perks. Don't forget about the perks.)

Till then, if you want some back patting for the good work you're doing, take a few trips around the office and fish for compliments from coworkers, who, thanks to rising estrogen, are far less annoying. Some are even downright tolerable. Or use your high-wattage writing skills to text message friends and brag about how your office would be just another casualty on F---edCompany.com without you.

Energy

Looking for some pep? Then you can save your money on that morning macchiato. You're getting a natural burst of energy from rising estrogen and testosterone that keeps you exhilarated, chatty, alert, and animated all day long. Good news if you have a hot date to go rock climbing tonight. Bad news if you're trying to convince your boss you're too tired to work another hour of overtime.

If you're sensitive to hormones, this power surge could be a bit too much to handle. You may feel anxiety, heart palpitations, or a racing pulse. And nervous habits, such as fidgeting, chewing your nails, or smoking, may increase. As you can imagine, caffeine, sugar, and other stimulants exaggerate these symptoms. So if you don't want to totally tweak out, avoid them altogether. Then again, if you get off on looking as twitchy as a backup dancer in an MC Hammer video, ask the espresso boy to pour you a double.

Diet

With testosterone rising, your sense of adventure in food is beginning to climb. It's not at fried blowfish levels just yet. But you are willing to attempt a new turkey chili recipe or risk a different flavor of Jell-O.

Day 4

Out of the Menstrual Hut

Mood

Grab your suitcase and pack up your Midol, heating pad, and aromatherapy candle. You've been voted out of the menstrual hut!

True, your period hasn't officially ended. You'll probably still be bleeding in dribs and drabs till tomorrow. But cramps are no longer gripping your innards like a cranky space being from one of those *Alien* movies. You're no longer so sapped of energy that simply opening a bag of Pepperidge Farm cookies leaves you too exhausted to work the remote. And whether your hormones are natural or you're taking hormone contraceptives, estrogen and testosterone rise to extrovert levels today. As a result, you no longer want the cloistered coddling that you'd craved since Day 27.[1]

So, like celebrities migrating home from their St. Bart's resorts after the first spring thaw, you're ready to emerge from hibernation—and there couldn't be a better time for it. You're feeling optimistic, confident, and energetic, which makes you fun to be around and, if you want it, the center of attention. So bask in your girly glory and throw yourself a coming out party!

Mind

Give it up for estrogen and testosterone. As they rise, they kick your brain into high gear. If only increasing your credit card limit was so easy.

Thinking

Remember the old days—like two days ago—when something as little as a ringing phone or a sneeze a block away was enough to make you lose your focus? No more. Your powers of concentration are enough to block out most distractions. Of course, probably not the really big ones, such as an elephant charging through the room or someone bringing a cake in to work.

As estrogen and testosterone rise, you're also thinking faster on your feet, absorbing new information easily, and making decisions a tad more quickly. If you don't want your boss to notice your sharper brain skills and give you more work, then be sure to throw a few more "dudes" into your sentences and have Tetris on your Web browser in case he gets any ideas.

Memory

You know that to-do list that's got, oh, 108 things on it just for today? Well, your memory is sharpening enough to remember at least half of it without looking. Tomorrow, it'll be sharp enough to remember why you still haven't gotten most of it done.

Verbal

How convenient—as your urge to chat surges, your speech is more fluent and you're experiencing far fewer verbal stumbles. Couldn't hormones do this same trick with your wallet—say, as your urge to spend surges, you experience much higher cash flow? Yeah right, that's probably as likely to happen as Martha Stewart ever landing in jail. Hey, wait!

The side of your brain highlighted today?

Right brain: At a time when you're feeling creative and you're in a more outgoing mood, you might just be tempted to get all imaginative about your social plans. If you do, you'll have the power to turn what might have been your default dinner/movie/drinks into a glitterati tailgate party of Tara Reid proportions. Okay, well, maybe not that big. You don't want to be in rehab by the end of the month.

Since Day 19 you've been introspective. But now as estrogen and testosterone rise, they have you taking more of an interest in other people—for instance, the secretive neighbor you suspect of being an international spy (more likely a file clerk with social anxiety disorder) and the coworker who steals everyone's snacks from the minifridge and thinks no one's onto her (not true: the trail of cupcake sprinkles leading to her desk was a total tipoff).

This is also the last day your sixth sense will be sharp. But you needn't worry, Mother Nature's not gonna leave you high and dry. In the coming days your other five senses sharpen and make up for the intuitive cross check. That way, if the sales guy is telling you something you're not sure you should believe—like that the frozen yogurt really only has two calories and zero fat—you'll be able to detect from the tone of his voice, the look in his eye, and the extra poundage on all the other frozen yogurt customers if it's the truth.

Romance

In a relationship . . .

You're conversational. You're upbeat. You're positively ravishing. Face it, you're excellent date material. But don't wait for him to make the first reservation. Use your testosterone-driven boldness to take matters into your own hands and call for a table at that swanky restaurant slash lounge that serves killer Godiva chocolate martinis, sign up for paired pampering at a day spa that offers a seaweed wrap and gem therapy, or head off to Prada for doubles clothes shopping.

Just a pipe dream? Nah. You want to hit the town too much to let your guy wriggle out of the plans you're making for two.

If you're single . . .

Extroverted estrogen and testosterone are prying you away from the chat rooms and personals and are pushing you to find a mate in ways that get you out into the world, such as hitting a dance club, joining a coed yoga class, or bringing your picket sign to a political rally.

The guy who'll catch your eye is the one who's bearing concert tickets, an invite to a celeb-studded after-party, an itinerary for a Tahitian trip for two, or whatever else gets you away from the couch long enough for the butt trench in the cushions to pop back up.

Sex

Have sex on your mind? Boy howdy. Sexual fantasies are making your mind as crowded as an open bar. In the interest of full disclosure, you should know that these delicious daydreams are merely a ploy by your sneaky testosterone to get you turned on enough to climb into bed with your partner. But once you do, this hormone promises to make the experience totally worth it by increasing the sensitivity of your nipples and clitoris, making it easy to climax, and once reached, it's making your orgasm so intense, it'll inspire you to go for seconds.

Want to supersize your sex drive?

Sign up for a competitive event! Simply anticipating being in a competition increases libido-boosting testosterone by as much as 24 percent.[2] Best part? This testosterone trick works with any kind of competition—soccer, basketball, bowling, ice skating, marathon running, a bakeoff, or even competitive feng shui design!

Money

As long as it gets you out of the house today, estrogen and testosterone have you spending on practically anything. Movies, restaurants, day spas, department stores, monster truck rallies. Anything.

Career

If there's travel involved in your work, you're already packing your bags. No trips in your job description? Then you'll probably at least feel like recruiting the gals for an out-of-office lunch someplace fun. And with half-price drink specials.

If you opt to head out with your work buds, in between the usual who-did-what-with-whom-on-whose-desk-and-with-which-office-supply gossip, you might be tempted to brag about the many ingenious business ideas you've been dreaming up these past few high-creativity days. Once your colleagues recognize the sheer brilliance of your plans, they may try to persuade you to suggest them to the boss the minute you get back to the office. Thank them for their vote of confidence, but put off approaching the higher-ups till Day 6 when your verbal, cognitive, and memory skills sharpen enough to give the most convincing proposal.

Energy

Depending on your sensitivity to hormones, your energy is at a level that's, at best, alert and enthusiastic, at worst, nervous and a little tweaky. But no matter what your sensitivity, as estrogen and testosterone rise today you'll have the power and endurance to make it through a whole overworked day, drinks with the gals afterward, and at least two rounds of "Hotel California" before someone a tad less wasted pulls the plug on the karaoke machine.

Diet

Estrogen is at a level where you're still craving old faves. Testosterone is rising to the point where you want to venture into new flaves. Old faves? New flaves? Oh, what to do? What to do? Of course—put new twists on familiar foods! Usually go for pepperoni pizza? Jazz it up with pineapple and ham. A die-hard chicken souper all the way? Tempt your taste buds with some equally healthy Japanese miso soup. Pumpkin pie or bust? Bust out with a ramekin of pumpkin crème brûlée!

Day 5

Making Your Voice Heard

Mood

Yesterday you turned your focus to the world outside yourself. Now that you've had a chance to look around, you've got lots of opinions about what you see—politics, the networks' new season lineup, the latest in tooth bling. It seems as if nothing can escape your critical eye. That's because rising estrogen and testosterone are moving you toward the analytical left brain phase of your menstrual cycle, which makes you more apt to evaluate the people and events around you.[1]

What's more, estrogen's making you chatty and testosterone's making you bold, so trying to keep all your opinions to yourself is like trying to keep Marilyn Manson away from the Clinique counter.

This doesn't mean people should be worried that you're all complaint and no compliment. Truth is, rising estrogen and testosterone are continuing to buoy your cheerful, optimistic mood. So you're just as likely to dole out praise as you are criticism. Which is good news for at least half the folks you run into today. And that'll probably be a lot since increasing estrogen and testosterone make socializing sound like a lot more fun than kicking back by yourself with a microwave potpie at home.

Mind

You're just one day away from the big day—when estrogen and testosterone push your brain skills up to the Super-woman range of their monthly cycles. So, where once you were simply smarter than most men, tomorrow you will be reigning queen of all that is brain function. And today? You're thisclose.

Thinking

Your ability to concentrate is getting so strong, you're able to focus with ease on even the boring stuff, such as instruction manuals or whenever your boss opens his mouth. You'll also be absorbing new information faster than a dry-clean-only top absorbs spilled red wine. And you're quicker at making little decisions—such as choosing between the soup or the salad, or which pair of black shoes to wear with your new skirt (the pair with two straps and a bow or the pair with two bows and a strap?).

Memory

With your memory getting sharper by the day, no one's off the hook. You'll remember that your boy toy didn't fix the sink as he promised, you'll recall the twenty-five bucks your best friend hasn't paid back yet, and you'll realize that it's the day the hunky UPS guy comes, which means it's also the day to break out the extra-low hip-huggers.

Verbal

Chat-loving estrogen and testosterone are giving you the urge to call up friends and family, ask office chums out to coffee, and corner unsuspecting neighbors in elevators. But it's not as if you're totally bogarting the conversation. Your heightened interest in the world around you turns you into a veritable Barbara Walters as you ply everyone with questions, from what's going on in their lives and what they think of the latest issues in healthcare, to whether or not they believe the rumor that Ashton Kutcher's been putting the moves on Florence Henderson.

The side of your brain highlighted today?

Right brain: Creative right brain—we hardly knew ye. Break out the hanky and cue the tear. You'll be giving your right brain a sendoff tomorrow when estrogen and testosterone rise enough to push you into your rational left brain phase. Oh, don't worry, creativity won't go away completely. It's not as if at the stroke of midnight you won't be able to think up a clever screen name or doodle anymore. But your imagination will be pushed aside as logic takes center stage.

Till then, put down that bon voyage cake and put your ingenious right brain to work while you've still got it. Think up innovative solutions, produce breathtaking artistic masterpieces, or generate imaginative moneymaking ideas. No? Then at least get creative with the pizza toppings.

With estrogen and testosterone at out-on-the-town levels, you're interested in hashing out social plans. For instance, maybe you're thinking of showing up at your boyfriend's band gig, attending a girlfriend's birthday bash, or setting up a blind date between two friends who couldn't be more incompatible. No, they won't hit it off. But it does assure you follow-up cappuccinos with each to hear their side of the horror story. Bad girl! And yet it gets you out of the house two more times this month.

Romance

If you're in a relationship . . .

A new Xbox game. A voice-operated TV remote. A La-Z-Boy with built-in heat and massage. All ways to thank your sweetie for not copping to just how close he is to having his head explode at this estrogen-fueled chatty time of month. Oh, you may have your hunches, what with that deer-in-the-headlights look every time you start a new conversation. But it's so easy to mistake his clamming up for just good listening skills.[2]

There's another thing your poor communication-challenged boy will have to put up with if he wants to cash in on your testosterone-driven sex drive. Now that estrogen is making you more opinionated and testosterone is boosting your boldness, you want to be the one in your relationship who chooses when and where to go on dates.[3] Is there a movie he wants to see or a restaurant he prefers to go to? You'll painstakingly explain why your choices are better. Which he, of course, will agree with if only it will stop the onslaught of confusing words, words, words!

If you're single . . .

With testosterone increasing your sense of adventure, you're thinking outside the bar for ways to meet someone new. Like hanging around the men's section at Macy's. Or entering fly-fishing competitions.

Sex

Like a virgin? Hardly. Not only are you making the first move, you're as tenacious as a sexual telemarketer. If one guy's not answering his cell, you're off speed dialing another. And for good reason: Your hormones are making sex thoroughly fulfilling. Rising estrogen has you lubricating at the first sign of arousal. Rising testosterone is making your nipples and clitoris sensitive. And orgasms are not only easy to reach, but so knee-knockingly intense you're answering the chocolate or sex question with, "Sex, definitely sex." Sorry, Godiva.

Want to supersize your sex drive?

Team up with your guy, then invite a couple over for game night. If you and your guy win, libido-boosting testosterone will surge 49 percent in you and a virility-enhancing 20 percent in him![4] If you lose, testosterone plunges in both you and your mate. So make sure you invite a couple you can easily beat!

Day 8 Day 9 Day 10 Day 11 Day 12 Day 13 Day 14

Money

Testosterone is pumping up your confidence in your finances and encouraging you to take risks with your money. "Go ahead, live a little," it purrs. "You deserve it."

Estrogen is assuring you that spending is all right. "It'll make you feel good. You won't have any guilt at all," it coos. And, hey, if the bills get too high, estrogen promises it'll get a part-time job and help out.

Now, you know estrogen can't get a job. (How would it even dress for an interview?) But you get sweet-talked by these two shop-loving hormones anyway.

Normally, this could spell disaster for your bank account. But lucky for you, as you transition into your more budget-conscious left brain phase, you're on the lookout for sales and discounts, which helps keep your spending in check. At least a little. Okay, you'll spend more than the annual budgets of most private universities. But you'll totally snag a great deal on that Hermès handbag.

Career

You're giving your opinions everywhere you go—in the boardroom, at meetings, by the water cooler, in the ladies room through the stall wall. Yak all you want. But put off proposing a new project or asking for a promotion or raise until tomorrow when confidence combines with skyrocketing verbal, cognitive, and memory skills to give an even more persuasive presentation.

If you've been letting others lead projects, assertiveness-inducing testosterone now has you piping up and persuading others to try it your way. Especially if their way hasn't gotten results. If your coworkers are wise to the ways of hormones and know how sharp estrogen and testosterone are making your brain functions, they'll happily appoint you team leader. Especially if their bonus check rides on the project's success. Otherwise, you may just have to wrest control by challenging them to a duel. Or a tongue-twister contest. With estrogen-fueled verbal skills on the rise, you're sure to totally cream them!

Energy

Your neighbor ask you to babysit? Your girlfriend need help moving? Your boyfriend looking for an extra hand while building the new entertainment center? You only wish you could claim exhaustion. But your animated expressions, chattiness, and Backstreet Boy–like bounce all give you away and reveal just how much pep rising estrogen and testosterone are giving you today.

Are you sensitive to hormones and have been experiencing anxiety or a racing pulse as a result of the recent estrogen and testosterone-fueled energy boost? These symptoms will likely subside by today as your body gets used to the upward climb, making it a smooth ride all the way up to the high-energy top on Day 13.

Diet

Loves-to-try-different-things testosterone is rising enough to make you yearn for new flavors—but it has not yet risen enough to go for the untried and untested. You'll be happiest with twists on old faves, such as salmon Caesar salad instead of your usual chicken, pancakes with blueberry syrup in place of your usual maple, or toast smothered in pecan apple butter rather than your usual margarine.

Counting fat grams, carbs, or calories? As you transition to your left brain phase, it's easier to recall the benefits of sticking to "allowed" foods, which makes it easier to deny yourself forbidden treats. Which means your roommate can now stop hiding her Nutella and Oreos underneath her laundry hamper. What? As if you weren't going to look there?

Health

Rising estrogen is making you forget all about those aches and pains from your low hormone days. And, as it continues its increase, it puts a positive spin on other health issues as well:

- If you suffer from asthma, arthritis, diabetes, depression, or epilepsy, your symptoms may improve today as estrogen rises.[5]
- Need a mammogram? Schedule one for between Days 5 to 12. Studies show that mammograms detect cancer more effectively on these days in premenopausal women.[6]

Switch to the Left Brain

Mood

Something important happens today. A one-day sale at your favorite boutique? Women's shoe designers admit they own stock in corn and bunion pads? Blue is declared the new brown?

Even more important: Estrogen and testosterone rise just enough to complete the shift from your creative and intuitive right brain phase to your logical and analytical left brain phase.[1] This means for the next fourteen days, emotions will take a back seat to reason, romantic idealism will make way for practicality, and hunches and gut instinct will be replaced by trips to the library and Google searches.

Yet, make no mistake—being a Rational Rita doesn't turn you into a total square. Hardly! Truth is, you're more adventurous than ever. Okay, so you're not getting your nipple pierced and flashing it for *Girls Gone Wild*. (That doesn't happen till Day 11.) But from today till Day 10, estrogen and testosterone are moving you in a decidedly bolder direction. For instance? Well, you might be tempted to hop a Vespa and cruise to Burning Man, run for political office, or answer an ad looking for backup dancers for Beyoncé's new video.

Your optimism, confidence, and ability to come up with insightful opinions that make any conversation more interesting are still going strong. In fact, these continue to increase right up to Day 13, making it a perfect time to schedule a party, attend a reunion, or show up at any other major social event where you want to reduce the women to jealous snipes and make the men sorry they didn't arrive solo.

Take hormone contraceptives? Then by now your hormones will have likely kicked in. What your estrogen and testosterone will be like for the rest of the month depends on which contraceptive you take:

If you take progesterone-only contraceptives (such as the mini-Pill or Depo-Provera), your estrogen and testosterone follow an up-and-down pattern that's similar to natural hormones.

If you take monophasic hormone contraceptives that contain both estrogen and progesterone (such as the pill, Ortho Evra patch, NuvaRing, Lunelle, or Seasonale, or if you use Depo-Provera along with an estrogen add-back therapy), estrogen and progesterone are doled out in a constant dose for the rest of the month. However, many women report that they still feel cyclical changes in their hormones. Some researchers believe it's because other body hormones and chemicals still follow cyclical monthly patterns. Other researchers believe it's because your own natural hormones break through. Either way, your estrogen and testosterone will be at elevated levels for the rest of the month. They probably just won't climb as high or fall as low as natural hormones.

If you take the biphasic or triphasic pill, estrogen is doled out in a constant amount, but progesterone rises throughout your cycle. So while your estrogen and testosterone may not climb as high or fall as low as natural hormones, your progesterone will follow a course similar to natural hormones.

Mind

Good news—your brain skills make the shift to the smart Superwoman phase of your menstrual cycle today! Want even better news? Estrogen and testosterone continue to make these brain skills improve all the way through to Day 13! Sound like eight amazing days you totally want to be a part of? You may address all fan mail to EstrogenandTestosterone@yourbod.com.

Thinking

Sure, your ability to concentrate and absorb new information are both strong today. But what's really worth talking about is that today through Day 10, estrogen and testosterone are at the exact levels you need to make the best choices possible,[2] testosterone has you picking a choice more quickly, and once you pick a plan of action, you have more conviction in it so you're less likely to change your mind. Meanwhile, estrogen has you feeling optimistic about the outcome, which means you're willing to take a riskier path if it feels like the right one. And now that both hormones have ushered in your logical left brain, it's easier to analyze options and you're more likely to base your decision on facts rather than emotions.

So what happens if you miss this Day 6 to Day 10 window for optimal decision making? Well, your life probably won't be thrown into complete chaos and no one will force you to watch *The Simple Life* as punishment. But there are pitfalls that make the other days less than perfect for making an important choice. For instance, on . . .

Days 11 to 13: Feelings of overconfidence from high testosterone can have you rushing to a decision before taking time to examine the facts. And that could lead to disaster, like buying a car that turns out to be a lemon or sniping a faux zebra stripe skirt off eBay before realizing it goes with nothing in your faux leopard skin wardrobe.

Days 14 to 28: Plunging estrogen and testosterone will be decreasing your self-confidence and coloring your decision with doubt. This could lead to lots of missed opportunities. For instance, you might not go for a plum job because you didn't think you had a shot. Or you might turn down an invite to be an MTV *Real World* housemate because you were afraid of the stigma it would have on you forever. Okay, well, that fear would probably be valid. But you get the point.

Days 20 to 28: You'll be in your emotional right brain phase and more likely to base your choice on feelings rather than logic, the facts, or what's most practical. This could lead to picking the hydraulic pumping low-rider over the more sensible Ford Focus, or splurging your savings on a weekend at an exclusive resort spa instead of investing it in a more practical four-year-college degree.

Days 1 to 5: Estrogen and testosterone may be on the rise, but they haven't risen to the high-confidence levels you'll need for the really major decisions, for instance, whether to change careers or to get bangs.

Of course, if an instant choice—submitting an offer on a house or agreeing to host the Emmys—is called for on any day, simply being aware of the limitations of each phase can help you overcome them.

Memory
Absent-mindedly putting your car keys in the fridge? As if. Staring at the ice cream on the supermarket shelf for thirty minutes trying to remember which flavor you like best? The dairy manager with the hots for you only wishes. Forgetting the name of the hottie who just introduced himself? Puhleeze, that's so Day 1. Today your memory is sharp, and only getting sharper as estrogen continues to rise.

Verbal
Chatty? Absolutely. Tongue-tied? Not a chance. You're verbal fluency is getting so good, you can even say "Which

wristwatches are Swiss wristwatches?" without stumbling. Okay, well, maybe on your third try. Okay, well, even if you still can't, you totally have that whole "Peter Piper picked a peck of pickled peppers" thing down. You can take another stab at the Swiss wristwatch line again on Day 13 when estrogen—and verbal fluency—are at their highest.

The side of your brain highlighted today?

Left brain: It's that time of month again—when practicality pushes aside creativity, logic replaces intuition, focusing on the world outside yourself is more interesting than scrutinizing your own thoughts and emotions, and you prefer to work in an organized space rather than one that's full of Post-It notes and messy piles. Sound like a big ol' bore? Don't worry—estrogen and testosterone are also pushing you to be increasingly daring and fun all the way through Day 13.

Romance

If you're in a relationship . . .

Love has so many metaphors to define it. An arrow straight through the heart. A red, red rose. A princess-cut diamond the size of Rhode Island.

Well, today yours is an airplane on autopilot. What the hay? Relax, it doesn't mean you're no longer working on your relationship to make it great. It just means you're too busy making out with your guy to have to bother with the controls.

And that's what your relationship will be about all the way till Day 13. Estrogen has you overlooking problems and issues you've had with your mate. And testosterone increases the secure feeling that you and your boy-toy will be together for the long haul. These hormones combine to make your relationship feel like such a smooth flight that you don't need to be in the pilot seat keeping it on course. You're just enjoying the ride.

If you're single . . .

Guys who catch your eye are those who have you chasing them. That's because testosterone is making the hunt for a hottie a total thrill. Thought only men hunted and that women gathered? Don't believe all the pictures you see drawn on cave walls. Gals hunt plenty: You hunt down bargains, you hunt down the last chocolate fudge brownie Ben & Jerry's, you hunt down the cat when it's time to go to the vet. You are an expert hunter. The only difference between you and a man is that you don't stuff your prey and display it in the den; you marry it and make it move furniture and do heavy lifting for you.

Sex

Testosterone is doing all it can to get you into bed: It's planting naughty thoughts in your mind when you're trying to do even the most unsexy activities, from tweezing chin hairs to ordering cheese fries. It's making you aroused by a man's scent and the feel of his hard, muscular chest when you "accidentally" bump up against him at the laundromat, in the elevator, and wherever else you can manage to corner him. And when your guy touches you, you could swear that your nerve endings have somehow all been hooked up straight to your lusty parts.

Once you cave to the carnal pressure, testosterone promises to make every minute spent canoodling worth it. It's increasing the sensitivity in your nipples and clitoris, has you easily reaching climax, and is working overtime to make your orgasms even more intense than in past days. "How's that even possible?" you might ask. "By radiating the sensation of your orgasm over more of your body," testosterone answers with a sinful grin. The result is an orgasm with such all-over intensity and power that you might just feel like Dr. Bruce Banner transforming into the Hulk. Only prettier. And, you know, not as green.

Are you and your guy in synch?

If you and your mate have been together for two or more years, then his testosterone level has synched up with yours.[3] No lie! As your testosterone rises over the course of your menstrual cycle, so does his. As your testosterone falls over the course of your menstrual cycle, his does, too. This means on Days 17 and 18 when both your testosterone levels are dipping, you'll be turning to each other in bed at the same time and saying, "Not tonight, dear. Jinx, owe me a Coke!"

53

Money

Free-spending testosterone has you whipping out your credit card with the frequency of Joan Rivers at a plastic surgery convention. But you're not totally off the hook with your wild splurging. With your analyzing left brain now in full gear, you're automatically keeping a mental tally of just how much you're buying. And the higher the tab goes, the higher the worry over how much you're shelling out. Appease both your shopaholic testosterone and spendthrift left brain by heading for the sales rack and hunting around for bargains. Or at least skip the in-store coffee bar that seems to always add another $60 to your shopping trip.

Career

When you were a kid, you probably pictured grown-up life as a time free of such things as groveling to your parents to get your allowance increased by, say, a quarter or begging to be trusted with more responsibility for, say, a goldfish.

What a drag it is to then discover that adult life isn't much better. There are no bosses strolling around the office with the sole purpose of seeking out hard-working employees to grant raises to. No supervisors recognizing your dependability and trustworthiness all on their own and asking you to take over the department.

No, it all comes down to the groveling and begging you, thankfully, honed in your youth.

Lucky for you, from today till Day 10, estrogen and testosterone reach levels that give you the best chance of hearing a yes for any of your requests. That's because these two hormones are giving you energy, optimism, and confidence that infuse you with a go-for-it attitude. On top of that, they're fitting you with the verbal and cognitive skills you need to present the most persuasive case and to handle any curve ball your boss throws at you.

Is your boss a guy? Then use *his* hormones to improve your chances of getting what you want. How so? Approach him in the late afternoon when his testosterone plummets, making him less likely to challenge your request.[4] Approach him any sooner and his aggressive high testosterone is more likely to make your request toast.

Want to give yourself an even bigger shot at hearing a yes from your boy boss? Then rein in all that estrogen- and testosterone-fueled talkativeness.[5] Men don't like to hear lots of words. And male supervisors like them even less. Oh, he'll tell all the other boy bosses that he hates a chatty Cathy because it makes her look ditzy. But the truth is, words easily make him confused and talking figure-eights around him doesn't help the situation any. So help him feel more secure by limiting the number of bon mots you say to him, let him talk without interrupting him, and when you answer, get straight to the point.

While you're at it, speak more s-l-o-w-l-y and make your voice sound deeper. Estrogen and testosterone are speeding up your speaking pace and raising the pitch of your voice.[6] Normally no biggie. But when dealing with men on the job, it's a totally different story. That's because men's minds are wired to read fast, high voices as flaky and read slow, deep voices as authoritative and intelligent.[7] Want proof? Look no further than politicians, voice-over actors in pharmaceutical commercials, and every celebrity who ever faced a judge. They all use this slow and low trick to make even their most dubious claims sound utterly convincing.

Having trouble reaching a lower pitch without sounding as though you're doing a Barry White imitation? Try lowering your chin a little. This should give you a deeper sound without that cartoon effect that can undermine your power- and smarts-enhancing image.[8]

Didn't muster your nerve to ask for a raise or promotion today? You've got until Day 10 to pipe up. Wait till Day 11 to 13 and high estrogen and testosterone may give you too much nervous energy, making you too talkative or hyper during your delivery. After Day 13, not only will the shine come off your verbal and cognitive abilities, making it harder to convince your boss, but you may be tempted to disclose exactly what you think of him and his lousy low-paying company should he turn you down.

Energy

Here's a cruel twist: On the days caffeine doesn't sap the last of your iron or make PMS worse, you don't even need it. Estrogen and testosterone are making you plenty zippy without any help from the whatever-cino you usually blow your rent money on.

Diet

Rising testosterone has you venturing out to find new flavors. This makes you want to try out different restaurants, spicier foods, and foreign cuisine . . . but not too foreign. Testosterone won't have you up for dishes like Nepalese Chhwela Wala till Day 11. For now, it has you preferring more common other-country fare—such as French, Italian, Indian, or Mexican.

On the Atkins, South Beach, or Subway diet? During your left brain phase you've got more conviction to steer clear of foods on your no-no list, even when your cubicle mate chows down on a whole box of Hostess Snoballs right in front of you. Then again, that's probably more of a deterrent to junk food than an enticement. And maybe even grounds for a cubicle transfer.

Day 7

Girls Just Wanna Have Fun

Mood

Party animal estrogen is turning you into a gal with can-can-do written all over her. You want to have fun. You want to frolic. You want to wake up with your underwear on your head and the vague memory of celebrities, flying acrobats, and some hot guy licking instant pudding off your chest.

Meanwhile, adventure-craving testosterone is pushing you to take risks, albeit calculated ones. This emboldening hormone doesn't have you flying on a trapeze without a net just yet, so you're still taking necessary precautions. For instance, you won't go jumping right off the bridge with that bungee rope tied around you; you'll make sure that the plungers on line ahead of you return with their skulls intact first. And, you won't leap right up on the fashion runway with a protest sign that reads **FUR BELONGS TO ITS ORIGINAL OWNER**; you'll make sure the color of your lettering coordinates with your outfit first.

Whatever it is you decide to do, make it exciting. Estrogen and testosterone have you craving action and new experiences. So save the open mic poetry for Day 23 when misery loves company. And open mic poetry.

Day 8   Day 9   Day 10   Day 11   Day 12   Day 13   Day 14

Estrogen's stressful side effect

Turns out, along with a sunny mood and optimistic outlook, estrogen also amps up your stress response from today through Day 13.[1] This could transform the minor anxiety you'd normally have over usual boot-shaking events—such as meeting your boyfriend's parents, giving a presentation at work, or taking a major test—into a total tummy-churning, sweat-soaking stress-out. Beat estrogen-induced stress with relaxation techniques such as yoga, meditation, or simple deep breathing.

Mind

Estrogen and testosterone continue to sharpen brain skills, make you chatty, and push you further into a logical phase. Now if only they could pay off all your school loans. Then they'd be perfect!

Thinking

It's easy to concentrate, you're absorbing new information quickly, and you're making the best decisions and have the most conviction in your choices. At this point, the only question left is what can't you do? (Besides turn back time and tell Halle to say no to *Catwoman*, that is.)

Memory

Okay, seriously, the fact that your memory is getting so good that you can spit out all the info you just heard in a five-hour meeting without even checking your notes plus recall all five names of the Jackson brothers is getting just a little intimidating.

Verbal

You're the conversationalist of every blind date's dreams—you're eloquent, can instantly find the exact words you're looking for, and have so much to say that all he practically has to do is sit there and look pretty. Oh, and pick up the check.

The side of your brain highlighted today?

Left brain: You're logical, practical, and full of wise decisions. You're like Alan Greenspan. Only funner!

With your focus on the world outside yourself, you're likely turning on the news, flipping through the latest *Entertainment Weekly*, and sending out bulk e-mails in search of juicy gossip.[2]

Romance

If you're in a relationship . . .

Flashback to the early days: He'd take you dancing, snorkeling, parasailing, extreme rock climbing on The Nose of El Capitan. Anything to prove he'd be the daring and courageous warrior of your dreams.

Today: The only adventure he sees is hunting down the remote, which he perpetually accuses you of hiding. (Okay, you did it. But without this fifteen-minute living room rampage would he get any exercise at all?)

Thing is, excitement-loving estrogen and testosterone still want to do all the fun, crazy activities of your courtship phase—especially from today to Day 13 when they're at their highest levels.

Your guy chickening out while you go ahead and sky-dive over the coast of Torquay? Go-it-alone testosterone is pumping up your feelings of independence so you're okay with him watching you from the ground while he holds your purse. [3] The really big pink one.

If you're single . . .

Lads with second-base appeal are those who are easygoing and don't want anything too serious. With have-fun-or-die-trying estrogen this high, you're in no mood to fix an emotional train wreck or constantly reassure a sentimental codependent who's bringing you stuffed teddy bears with notes that say "I ❤ you 4ever" after your very first date. [4]

$\int e^x$

You know how you hear a commercial with a catchy jingle and you just can't seem to get it out of your head for the rest of the day? Well, sex is like that jingle—you just can't seem to shake it. Brushing your teeth? You'll be thinking of sex. Watching the weather channel? Thinking of sex. Driving by roadkill? Yup, here comes sex again.

That's testosterone's fault. It's simply trying to remind you that if you take time out for sex or masturbation, it'll make it worth missing *Scrubs* for. And with any luck, *ER*, too. That's because testosterone has you getting aroused quickly, is making your nipples and clitoris sensitive to touch, and climax easy to reach. And, once reached, your orgasm is so intense, you'll probably feel like you'll never have one like it again. (Not true. Testosterone packs a climactic punch clear through to Day 15.)

With estrogen and testosterone reaching adventure-loving levels, you may feel the urge to mix things up today through Day 13. Perhaps you'll consider new positions, want to try out new locations, or experiment with battery-operated toys that come in three speeds. Whatever you propose, have patience with your guy. He's still trying to figure out how to make you orgasm the regular way. Introducing untested maneuvers may be intimidating and make him feel less like a superstud in the sack and more like a bull in a vagina shop.

Money

Splurge-happy estrogen and testosterone are urging you to spend as if the state of the economy depended on your buying those strappy sandals. But your analytical left brain continues to urge you to be practical about your finances and—horrors—find ways to save.

Oh, which influence to follow? Which influence to follow? Why not follow both by spending on items that will save you money? Order a credit report. Buy budgeting software. Purchase a receipt folder. Anything that helps you gain control over your finances. That way, when confidence about money decreases from Day 14 to Day 28, you won't feel so broke that you need to pick up moonlighting work doing something that totally goes against your morals and makes you feel really dirty. For instance, being one of those fake moviegoers in TV ads who gush rave reviews about a film like *Gigli*. :::Shiver:::

Career

Didn't ask for that raise or promotion yesterday? Go for it today. Same goes for proposing a new project, your own column, or any one of the novel ideas you had during your high creativity phase of Days 20 to 5. Not only are your optimism, confidence, and energy soaring, but estrogen and testosterone have you thinking faster on your feet, handling every curve ball, and giving you a memory sharp enough to recall every reason why you deserve a yes.

Just remember to follow the most important rule when making a request to a male boss: Wait to approach him till late in the afternoon when his assertiveness-inducing testosterone takes a dive, making him much more open to giving you what you want.

During this estrogen-soaked phase, you're seeing the world as one opportunity for fun after another—and work is no exception. Okay, maybe not *work* work. But you are more interested in hanging out with colleagues for lunch, planning after-hours meet-ups, or inciting the troops to rebel against the no casual Fridays policy by handing out cutoff shorts and tube tops.

During the day, you'll probably feel as if you can't get started until you've cleaned up your desk and thrown away old files and papers. That's your left brain influence. It prefers to work in a neat, organized environment rather than among the piles from your right brain days.

Right brain estimating tendencies are also out during your left brain phase. Instead, you're checking the time more often and are on top of deadlines. You're also more successful if you start and finish one project at a time rather than use right brain multitasking. It won't be too difficult to switch work methods, though; testosterone is pumping up your powers of concentration, giving you more focus than a fourteen-year-old boy downloading a Pamela Anderson pic.

Energy

Estrogen and testosterone are boosting your energy and stamina to a level that makes it feel as though you can stay alert through the most hectic of days and still be able to mosh it up at a Linkin Park concert, crash the gig's after-hours party, suck face with what you hope was one of the band members, run to a twenty-four-hour drugstore to buy coverup for the legion of hickies polka-dotting your neck, and still be able to get to work on time in the A.M.

Feeling as though you're getting through tasks a lot faster today? It's not your imagination. Not only are rising estrogen and testosterone boosting your energy and endurance, they're making you perform faster on non-thinking tasks such as talking, walking, typing, and deleting any e-mail with the subject line that begins with "Pump up the size of your . . . "

Diet

Adventurous testosterone is pushing you to try new recipes. And estrogen is making your taste buds increasingly more sensitive to flavor. This is giving you a hankering for foods that you haven't had in a long while or that are slightly different from your usual routine.

Cutting out sugar, white flour, meat, or orange foods from your diet? You'll feel more determined to follow your restricted regimen during the left brain phase when it's easier to recall the reasons behind your meal plan.

Breast self-exam alert

With your breasts no longer swollen or tender, today is the best day to perform your monthly BSE, an important method for finding cancer in its early stages.[5]

Day 8

Break Out the Tiara

Mood

Let's review. Your booty is delicious-looking. A given. You're a social magnet who attracts everyone you meet. Of course. What's left to have? High optimism, booming confidence, an adventurous spirit. Check, check, check. What about the love? Are you getting the love? Time to do a spot check, because if there's one thing estrogen and testosterone have you ~~wanting needing~~ demanding today it's a little R-E-S-P-E-C-T.

And, seriously, why shouldn't you get it? You totally rock. You figuratively roll. You are the one they turn to when the chips are down or the cable goes out. So use your testosterone-driven boldness that's increasing by the day and command that friends, family, coworkers, and boyfriends acknowledge your diva worthiness and show the proper appreciation for the perfection that is you.

But getting the love doesn't stop with those around you. Estrogen and testosterone are also pushing your confidence up another rung on the how-kickass-am-I! ladder, and that has you marveling at your own greatness. You're smart. You're a riot to be around. And if you don't look like the women splayed out in Versace ads, who cares? With so much to offer, you can't even understand why any gal would fritter away her life trying to conform to what a horny frat boy finds attractive. You've got better things to do.

Such as? Such as how about everything! With estrogen and testosterone pumping up your sense of self-sufficiency, you're feeling more independent than a single, freelance, atheist orphan. So you don't want to wait around for friends or the boy toy to get the soirée started. You're content jetting around town by yourself doing your own thing. A cool art opening for a friend from college? You are so there. A craft fair downtown? You're bringing a table, a chair, and a bagful of your best macramés. Pie-eating contest with a $100 prize? You go just for the free pie. Now *that* deserves respect!

Slam the brakes on estrogen stress-outs!

Sniff your boyfriend's unwashed, undeodorized armpits. Yup, you read right. Unwashed. Undeodorized. Armpits. Turns out, the smell of a guy's sweat relieves tension and induces relaxation in women.[1] Researchers aren't exactly sure why it works. Though they are sure it's not due to the aroma, which pretty much rules out Eau de Sweaty Armpit hitting the shelves at Sephora anytime soon.

Mind

Your brain continues to get a boost from estrogen and testosterone, making these two hormones better than a whole freezer full of Ben & Jerry's ice cream. Yes, that good.

Thinking

Your powers of concentration, learning ability, and decision-making skills are sharp and getting sharper all the way through Day 13. So you may want to use this time to launch a new business, make your run for Congress, or work on a cure for that horrible disease that turns Mousketeers into vacuous pop stars.

Memory

When you call your boyfriend on not giving you a card for your quarter-year anniversary, he's going to wonder how you could've remembered a little detail like that.

Verbal

Woe to the telephone survey dude who gets your number today. Not only are you in the mood to spend two hours explaining why you prefer Goobers over peanut M&Ms, your verbal fluency and word recall are so high, you'll have lost him long before you got to how you can tell the difference in tensile strength between the two brands of chocolate-covered nuts.

The side of your brain highlighted today?

Left brain: Decisions are based on what's most practical, you're more curious about the world around you, and you prefer your space to be neat and organized. Sounds suspiciously adultlike. But don't worry—high estrogen's working overtime to lure you into some totally non-adult-like high jinks. So your street cred is safe.

Romance

If you're in a relationship . . .

It's not that you outright demand gratitude, but you may expect at least a little from your guy. After all, high estrogen and testosterone have you knowing that you are, indeed, a goddess. Your wit is incisive. Your charm effusive. Your beauty unrivaled. Hmm, maybe you should be demanding it after all.

Regardless of how much gratitude your lad shows, estrogen still has you feeling close to him and doing all those things that close couples do, such as noticing the same things, sharing inside jokes, and calling each other by those baby-waby nicknames that make everyone else around you gag. But you don't care. Every shared laugh and shmoopie-woopie makes you feel instantly more secure in your relationship.

If you're single . . .

Not-content-till-you-land-a-mate estrogen and testosterone are pushing you out into the world to find a man. And, just in case you forget to take time out for the hunt, they'll be reminding you throughout the day by planting various boy-snaring ideas into your head, such as slipping that hard-bodied bike messenger your digits, sending a flirtatious e-mail to the new guy in IT, or sending over a soy latté to that shaggy-haired dude who hangs out at your café but whose cute, little bespectacled nose is always frustratingly lodged in a Sartre book.

Sex

Here's a little fact: Among both married and unmarried couples, sex is most frequent on Day 8.[2] Here's another little fact: From start to orgasm, a man's average endurance time is around two and a half minutes; for a woman, the same average is thirteen minutes.[3]

Talk about a letdown. But, it's not all his fault. For most mammals, sex is a rapid-fire affair. In male chimpanzees, for instance, the whole tryst lasts a cry-yourself-to-sleep three seconds.

Why the biological gyp? The quickie evolved so that animals and cave couples could procreate before predators had time to attack.[4] But with most of Modern Man and Woman's predators now eaten into extinction, made into coats, or confined to zoos where they're kept in check by taunting gradeschoolers, your man has no more excuses.

Research (and Ron Jeremy) prove that even though your guy can be off in a shot, he can also hold off for much longer—for hours, in fact. So make use of your testoster-one-fueled assertiveness and tell him to wait for you. Or to at least be ready to go again if he can't. The rewards for piping up will be many since testosterone is increasing sensitivity in your nipples and clitoris, making it easier to reach orgasm, and making your orgasms so powerful and all-encompassing, you're pretty sure you would've risked being eaten by a saber-toothed tiger to have one.

Money

$10,000: the amount you think is in your bank. $57.50: the amount that's really there. Why the difference? Blame that cash-confident testosterone. It's pumping up the feeling that you've got money to burn. And spend-as-sport estrogen is no less to blame. It's making you feel like treating yourself to fun stuff regardless of the price.

The only budget-conscious part of your body that you've got watching over your bottom line right now is your analytical left brain. It's quietly keeping a tally of how much you're spending and is urging you to slow down—or at least look for a better bargain—when the ink flows from black to red.

Career

The dream job: High pay. Low stress. Lots of fun. *Your job:* Low pay. High stress. Fun only when that guy from accounting gets drunk at after-work parties and hurls all over his Dockers.

Are ever the twain to meet? Of course! Okay, probably not. But you can inch closer to the fantasy by using today's high confidence, verbal fluency, short-term memory, and cognitive skills to propose a new department, product, or project, or by going for the big cheese and asking for a raise or promotion. Making your request to a male boss? Then increase your chances of hearing that sought-after yes by approaching him late in the afternoon when his puts-up-a-fight testosterone takes a dive, leaving him in the passive pussycat phase of his daily cycle.

Even if you don't make any special requests of your supervisors today, sunny-side-of-the-street estrogen is still making even the worst-paying McJob seem more fun. Okay, more tolerable. All right, at least you won't be burning down the file cabinets and threatening to let a thousand mosquitoes loose in the boss's office. And that's because high estrogen is making work seem less stressful, clients easier to deal with, and coworkers more like compatriots instead of corporate plants hired just to irk you all day.

You may feel the urge from your organization-loving left brain to tidy up your work station and focus on one project at a time rather than multitask. You're also keeping your eye on the clock and being sensitive to deadlines. But you don't have to worry much about missing a cutoff since estrogen and testosterone are making you pick up the pace on lots of non-thinking tasks—such as typing, reading, filing, and flinging spitballs over your cubicle's half wall.

Energy

Your boss needs you to work overtime? Bring it on! On the same evening you have a date to go merengue dancing? No prob! On the same night you were going to train to qualify for the Olympic triathlon team? You don't even flinch. Not when estrogen and testosterone are pumping you full of this much endurance and energy.

Diet

Adventurous testosterone craves variety. And high estrogen is making your taste buds become increasingly more sensitive to flavor. Together, this puts you in the mood for something a tad left of center of your palate, such as garlicky tabouli, tangy raw oysters, or a plate of spicy-hot chicken vindaloo.

Are you flexitarian trying to convert to vegetarian? Or a vegetarian trying to graduate to veganism? You'll be better able to resist the temptation of eating anything that could have been a pet during your left brain phase, which makes it easier to recall the reasons behind your food conversion.

Day 9

You've Got the Power!

Mood

Self-help superguru Tony Robbins: an eight-foot-high giant with a set of choppers the size of the Grand Tetons. Sure he's got personal power—he can crush an incorporated village with a single jumping jack.

You: someone who doesn't need to look for empowerment in any of Tony Robbins's "programs." (Can't he just say "book" like everyone else?) That's because estrogen and testosterone are pumping up your feelings of personal power to the heights of corporate heads just before they're subpoenaed. You have a take-charge attitude that makes even the surliest waiter serve your food before it gets cold. Goals seem attainable, even in high heels. And you're taking control over every aspect of your life—emotions, finances, romance, career, the disaster that is your purse. Nothing can stop you![1]

But that's not all! In their quest to be voted "Favorite Hormones, Like, Ever," estrogen and testosterone amp up the good vibrations they've been sending your way since Day 1: You've got the confidence door-to-door vacuum salesmen would give their best three-easy-payment power nozzle for. The kind of sunny optimism that comprises every nucleotide of Kelly Ripa's DNA. And your inner socialite is working the room with more ease than Kristi Yamaguchi covered in Astroglide.

Slam the brakes on estrogen stress-outs!

Take a bubble bath! It'll relax you by boosting anxiety-busting endorphins and loosening tense muscles that contribute to stress.[2]

Mind

As estrogen and testosterone rise, they continue to make your brain skills even sharper. The odds-on favorite is that you are so loving your estrogen and testosterone right about now.

Thinking

You've got the pinpoint focus of an actor trying to escape from her management contract after finding she's been booked on *Celebrity Mole*, you're more information-absorbent than a nine-year-old overhearing you discuss your "secret" butt lipo, and you're making decisions with more ease than it takes to dis Carrot Top.

Memory

Your memory's getting so sharp, you're recalling names and facts with the clarity of a defendant with a rock-solid alibi. Or at least a personal assistant with a grudge, who blows the whistle on her boss.

Verbal

Saying you've got the urge to chat is like saying Kim Jung-Il has the urge to act a little wacky. But be warned: Flip that phone too much and by the end of the day you may need an ice pack for your aching elbow. If you do end up needing medical care, at least you've got your excellent verbal skills to explain to the doctor exactly what happened.

The side of your brain highlighted today?

Left brain: You're seeing life through a logical lens. Which doesn't mean you won't make some impractical decisions. You'll just be better at rationalizing them. Which may explain all those salad shooters from QVC.

Romance

If you're in a relationship . . .

Stand by your man? Yes. Wear your hair up just for him? Maybe. Give him control over the remote? Not ever! Well, at least not until Day 17, when low levels of estrogen and testosterone have you graciously letting him think he's making some of the decisions in your relationship once again—such as which TV shows to watch, where to go on dates, and what he'll be buying you for your anniversary. Till then high estrogen and testosterone have you pulling rank as the "better half" and insisting on your choice simply because it's your choice, and, well, because you have the vagina.

If you're single . . .

Pricey tuxes catch your eye. Private jets turn you to jelly. And an entire country bowing to his supremacy has you calling the wedding planner you've had on retainer since you were fifteen. Sensing a pattern here? The more power a guy displays, the sexier he becomes. The reason? Estrogen and testosterone have you on the hunt for the best provider for your adorable little ovum.[3] In the olden days, you would have jumped Grok, the lead caveman with the latest in fire-making tools. Today it's Donald, the billionaire real estate mogul with a bad comb-over and his own fleet of bulletproof BMWs.

Sex

If there's one thing on your mind today it's—well, okay, it's taking over the world. But if there are *two* things on your mind today, it's taking over the world and getting your boy—or toy—into bed. Give in to the carnal cravings and testosterone will repay you by helping you keep a tighter focus on your fantasies, making your nipples and clitoris sensitive to the slightest touch, and pumping up the sensation of your orgasms till they're even more intense than that tortured artist you dated in college.

Money

Aren't one of the lucky few who have a million-dollar trust fund? Then you may want to put a padlock on that purse. That's because free-spending testosterone is pushing you to buy, buy, buy! You're especially attracted to items that feed your sense of personal power—jewelry, designer labels, and a fourteen-bedroom manse in Southampton equipped with more maids' quarters than you can shake a Swiffer stick at.

With optimistic estrogen high, it feels as if you can really afford all these pricey luxuries. At least while you're handing over your credit card. But once you get back home, like an internal auditor, your budget-conscious left brain is off comparing your purchases against your checking account balance and setting off the panic alarm when the tally gets too high. Best to hold on to those receipts in case emergency returns are called for.

Career

You step into the office and something seems, well, different. You could swear that you spotted a starting line when you walked through the front door. You're pretty sure you hear the faint sound of a starter pistol coming from somewhere near Human Resources. And your coworkers—are they all wearing Nike running shoes?

Yes, but that's just because they haven't slipped into their toe-crushing heels yet. But they may as well be wearing sneakers all day now that competition-loving testosterone is high enough to make you feel as if you're in a race against your peers to the top.[4]

But what about all that estrogen-fueled love you've been feeling for your coworkers since Day 1? Oh, you're still feeling it. You've just now got to decide which influence to follow—cutthroat testosterone (which, by the way, will help get you that raise, promotion, and nifty ergonomic leather chair you've been eyeing in the office supply catalog) or the mushy, we're-in-this-together estrogen (that no doubt will make office parties more fun, but, let's face it, won't help pay off your student loans).

Sigh. What's an aspiring you to do? Perhaps suggest the team ask for an everyone-or-no-one, *Friends*-like raise during a group hug and see if it flies? Negative, Ghost Rider. Your mission is to make a bundle and get out before the corporate heads blow your 401(k) on strippergrams.

Is the fear that you can't pull off a straight win against your coworkers-cum-competitors holding you back? Relax. With estrogen and testosterone making your verbal, memory, and cognitive abilities sharp and the confidence in your talents soar, you're a personal power-filled force to be reckoned with.

On top of all that, this is still a prime time for approaching your boss about a raise, promotion, or that cool project you want to propose. And if you're asking a male supervisor, be sure to give yourself the competitive edge by holding off your request till late in the afternoon when his testosterone plummets, making him more open to saying yes.

Once you return from the boss's office, it's up to you to decide whether or not you want to use that estrogen- and testosterone-fueled energy to take a victory lap.

Energy

You've got the stamina of a filibustering senator. You're running around faster than an ADHD kid in need of Ritalin. And you're jumping over tall skinny mochaccinos in a single bound. What's responsible for this incredible power surge? Address all thank-you cards to energizing estrogen and testosterone.

Diet

On the menu today: Any off-the-eaten-path recipe that excites your adventure-loving testosterone and gives your increasingly sensitive taste buds a thrill ride. Fried blowfish and raw octopus are not totally out of the question.

On the all Kashi and granola diet? Your logical left brain is helping you resist the temptation to sneak your roommate's Count Chocula. His beef jerky collection, however, is totally safe.

Superstar!

Mood

High estrogen and testosterone have you trading up: Since Day 2 you've been optimistic; today you can see the silver lining even in the return of Hanson. Since Day 3 you've been confident; today you have less doubt than the Winona Ryder judge. Since Day 4 you've been outgoing. Today you're totally Nicole Richie.

You're also beginning to feel urges to be bold and experiment. That's adventure-loving testosterone's influence—as it gets closer to its peak on Day 13, it becomes like that pushy friend from high school who was always calling you chicken till you agreed to eat the glue / moon the basketball team / kiss that nerdy seventh grader who wore bow ties to school. It's egging you on to do pretty much anything daring and just a little outrageous. Oh, the impulses might start out slow—maybe try a new eye shadow color or change the ring tone on your phone. But pretty soon testosterone will have you tapping into your wild side and before you know it, you'll be eating the fried blowfish / baring your breasts at the Mermaid Parade /

kissing that seventh grader who, thankfully, grew up to be a sharp-dressing Wall Street bond trader with a house on the Cape.

Slam the brakes on estrogen stress-outs!

Ask your honey to give you a massage. It'll relax you by pumping up anxiety-busting endorphins and decreasing cortisol that contributes to stress![1]

Estrogen's hidden risk

From today through Day 13, high estrogen makes you more likely to get hooked on cigarettes, cocaine, and other addictive substances.[2] Suffice to say, you're better off saving the Cinnabons till Day 14 when the risk of getting strung out on them decreases.

Mind

Rising estrogen and testosterone just keep right on fueling your stellar brain skills. If only your morning Coolatta was this effective.

Thinking

No superchip implanted in your brain. No direct link to Deep Blue. No Stephen Hawking on speed dial. At this point, your friends and coworkers are wondering just how you can have such stellar focus, decision-making skills, and learning ability without outside help.

Memory

Orange. 148. Uvula. Your memory is getting so sharp, you're recalling the answers you gave on your fifth-grade biology test. And even the ones you peeked at from the girl sitting next to you.

Verbal

Just think—if David Bowie had the amazing verbal powers you have today, he never would have famously stuttered "Ch-ch-ch-ch-changes." Then again, stuttering was pretty big back then. Why else would Roger Daltry have exalted "my g-g-generation"? Good thing they got that diction thing cleared up once grunge came along.

The side of your brain highlighted today?

Left brain: You tend to base your decisions on research or what's most practical. The results aren't as interesting as, say, basing it on your emotions or consulting your tea leaves. But then again, you're not stuck with a gallon of mugwort or a plynyl miniskirt either.

You have a deeper interest in the world outside your own, which makes you peek at the paper for the latest news, turn to *E!* for the hottest celeb sightings, and hit the knitting circle phone tree to catch up with your buds.

Day 1 Day 2 Day 3 Day 4 Day 5 Day 6 Day 7

Romance

If you're in a relationship . . .

Estrogen and testosterone have you feeling close to your mate and overlooking problems in your relationship. But these hormones are also making you feel too super sexy, confident, fun, and outgoing not to flirt up a storm with other guys.[3] So you do, with just about every guy you see. Even those you shouldn't? Including your roommate? The pizza guy? And your married personal trainer? Nooooo. Okay, yes. But it's all right because your excellent verbal abilities enable you to gracefully back out if you get in too deep.

If you're single . . .

The guys who catch your eye today are those who shower you with gifts, are physically strong and healthy, and have personal power. A job (and some bling bling) doesn't hurt either. Except for the job part, this sounds a lot like Mr. T. But don't worry, your hormones aren't trying to set you up with aging action stars with unfortunate hair. High estrogen is simply making you attracted to guys who are potential baby-daddy material and who look as if they can afford to keep the kid in pricey diapers till toilet training.

Sex

Estrogen and testosterone are making the confidence you have in your sexiness hit überlevels. Got a few extra pounds? So what. No one's kicking Queen Latifah or Mia

Tyler out of bed. Got a bad dye job? No prob. Green hair brings out the blue in your eyes. Got drunk one night and tattooed "I ❤ Derek Jeter" on your forehead? Big deal. Yankee fans will love you even more.

Know what else? Your guy thinks you're pretty sexy, too. In fact, researchers found there's a direct link between the depth of affection he has for you and how hot he thinks you look. Meaning? Meaning if he digs you, it'll melt inches off your thighs and tummy, iron out facial wrinkles, and fill in butt dimples without a single collagen injection. But if you have a bad 'tude, even if you're the most physically stunning woman alive, he's gonna think you're about as attractive as Leatherface.[4] Think of it as "love specs," the more respectable cousin of beer goggles. (And a fitting biological "In your face!" to snarky supermodels.)

Once you get sexy you into the bedroom, estrogen and testosterone are making lovemaking and masturbation a more thrilling ride than Disneyland's Thunder Mountain. Estrogen is keeping you lubricated with every twist and turn, which makes sex more comfortable and, therefore, more pleasurable. Testosterone is making you quick to be aroused, your nipples and clitoris sensitive to touch, and your orgasms more breathtaking than that first roller coaster dip. And both hormones are improving concentration, which makes it easier to ignore those annoying, little noises that can be so distracting—for instance, the phone ringing or the neighbors yelling through their floor at you to keep it down. That way, you can focus on the important stuff, like your body, your guy, or the fantasies propelling you like an out-of-control roller coaster car toward climax.

Money

Sigh. If only you were an heiress born with an Amex Black Card in your mouth. Oh well, at least you can still shop like one. Spend-it-like-you-got-it testosterone is building up your confidence to buy items that are so out of your price range. And don't-worry-be-happy estrogen is promising to assuage any guilt over the costly expenditures. To make things even more enticing, the excitement from high estrogen and testosterone is beginning to outweigh your logical left brain that's been (barely) keeping your checkbook in check these past few days. The result is a powder keg of splurging that threatens to make your credit card balance climb like the deficit.

Purchases that appeal most to you today are (surprise, surprise) big buys, such as a new computer, car, or maybe even that small island off the coast of Florida that's for sale on eBay. You're also attracted to items that boost your personal power, like the latest high-tech gadget that fits conveniently in your Fendi bag and which you can whip out the moment a VIP (Very Impressionable Person) walks by.

Career

Word has it that something important happens at work today. Is it that the guy in charge of supplies dares to replace your multicolored paper clips with cheaper— and far less cute—metallic ones? Or that the temp from accounting finally admits he's the one stealing everyone's lunch out of the fridge? Or that your most difficult client sends roses and a note apologizing for chewing you out about your company's choice of on-hold music?

Nope, something even more important. Today is the final day that estrogen, testosterone, and your left brain perfectly combine to make you as well-spoken as an Aaron Sorkin character and more persuasive than a Sally Struthers sponsor-a-child pitch.[5] And that's exactly what you need to help snag that raise, promotion, or green light for your pet project.

Wait for tomorrow through Day 13 to approach the boss and overexcited estrogen and testosterone could make you look too antsy or hyper (OK, flaky) to be considered higher tax bracket material. But if you wait until Day 14 to Day 5, you'll miss out on the estrogen and testosterone-boosting confidence that makes you fearless and feel not one bit like backing down at the first sign of a no.

In fact, the only time you should be waiting today is if your boss is a guy. In that case, put off your request till late in the afternoon. That's when his testosterone level takes a dive, making him less likely to find a reason to deny your request and more likely to see the wisdom in giving you want you want.

Even if you don't have any plans to ask for extras from your boss, you're still working harder at your job today. That's because high testosterone is turning you into a competitive overachiever who wants to prove to the higher-ups that you can one day take over the company. Or at least make them afraid that you'll soon be their biggest competitor so they should pay you more to keep you from putting them out of business.

Energy

You know all that zest and endurance that have been steadily building up since Day 1? That was just the warmup act. Now you're so pumped it feels as if you've got Red Bull being piped in through a central vein. What's more, your energy and stamina remain this high through Day 13. So if you had some particularly strenuous activities you were putting off for a more energetic day—say, piloting a catamaran around the Fiji Islands or plowing a few hundred acres of farmland by hand—you've got no more excuses.

Diet

Inspired by will-try-anything-once testosterone, your tongue is packing its bags and setting sail for distant lands. Whether you come along or not is your decision. But if you want to catch up with it, you can find it sampling a little asa kitfo at the Ethiopian restaurant, tasting a bit of Norwegian smoked salmon at the fish market, and indulging in a decadent Belgian chocolate mousse at the gourmet bakery.

Cutting out all sugar from your diet? Restricting yourself to only blue foods? Whatever your limitations, it's easier to stick to them with your left brain doling out conviction in heaping side dishfuls.

Gossip Page Days

Mood

Why has being sensible and levelheaded gotten such a bum rap? Sometimes it's just the thing. For instance, you should always act blasé when your publicist introduces you to her celebrity clientele. Keep your cool when coming face-to-face with your ex-boyfriend and his new flame. And throwing your panties onstage during a Yo-Yo Ma concert is definitely a gentlewoman no-no.

Why it's gotten such a bum rap, obviously, is that it's a total drag. How much more fun it would be if you were, say, the mystery girl canoodling with a movie star in the blind item on Page Six. The Charlize look-a-like that paparazzi snapped outside a dance club duking it out with Shannen Dougherty. Or the woman found by security hiding out in Sting's dressing room wearing nothing but a "Yoga is for lovers" thong and a tantric smile.

So maybe it's a good thing that risk-taking testosterone and optimistic estrogen hit *Thelma & Louise* heights today.[1] That way, you'll be more likely to give in to fearlessness and passion rather than settle for plain ol' politeness and dreary decorum.

Do you take hormone contraceptives that dole out a constant amount of estrogen? Then your estrogen won't reach the high level that natural hormones do, which means you're also less likely to reach the lampshade-on-head level of outrageousness that natural hormoned gals achieve. Oh, you're still up for a daring good time. You'll just have fewer compromising Polaroids pop up when you make your run for Congress.

Regardless of whether your hormones are natural or you're taking hormone contraceptives, you'll likely enjoy whatever parties you can manage to crash and whatever high jinks you can convince your lower-hormoned friends to join you in. That's because estrogen and testosterone are keeping you upbeat and confident. Even being captured in the eyes closed, mouth open paparazzi shot of every woman's nightmare doesn't faze you. You just marvel at how your blue eye shadow really brings out the sparkle in your teeth.

But make no mistake—this hormone-fueled happiness doesn't mean you're all Katie Couric sweetness and light. Get you in a high-stakes round of Pictionary or Jenga and competition-loving testosterone will turn you into a cutthroat contestant who's tempted to stoop to Tonya Harding levels to win. Keep a box of Kleenex around for thin-skinned friends who mistakenly believed they were in for a fun time at game night.

Slam the brakes on an estrogen stress-out!

Go for a walk, hit the gym, pull the dirty laundry off the exercise bike and pedal away for a while, or do any other kind of workout you can think of. Research shows that exercise is a top way to pump up anxiety-busting endorphins!

Mind

With estrogen and testosterone continuing to rise and making your brain skills even sharper, what's not to love about Day 11?

Thinking

Quick—what is it that you want to do that requires intense concentration, the ability to absorb new information at light speed, and split-second decision making? Whatever it is, you've got today through Day 13 to get it in while high estrogen and testosterone make you as brainy as you're going to be all cycle.

Memory

Your powers of recall are so strong you probably think you can auction off your PDA on eBay. Don't let it get to your head. You're going to need that electronic reminder again by the time Day 23 rolls around, when you'll be wondering how you ever got by without it.

Verbal

Eloquent, recalls words easily, an engaging conversationalist. Is this you or an ad for a TV talk show host? It's you. But if you answer an ad for talk show host today, chances are you'll totally snag it.

The side of your brain highlighted today?

Left brain: With high estrogen pushing you to release your inner wild child, it may sometimes be difficult for others to believe that you're actually viewing the world through a more logical and practical lens.

Romance

If you're in a relationship . . .

Estrogen and testosterone are making your relationship tight, your feelings toward your mate loving, and all his faults as forgettable as *Blair Witch 2*.

So why is your eye on the *other* guy?

For starters, estrogen and testosterone are giving you the confidence to believe you're a total knockout and are revving up your libido to *Sex and the City* levels. That's like giving you a backstage pass to a Red Hot Chili Peppers concert and immunity to STDs.

What's more, it's estrogen and testosterone's job to urge you to take another look around to make sure you're choosing the right guy to fertilize your ovum. Is the guy you're already with healthy? Strong? A genetic donor with DNA appeal? Your hormones still seem to think it's worth another look-see just to make sure there's not someone better.

Can't resist sneaking a peek even when your lad's around? Relax. Your guy will be none the wiser. While a man needs to conspicuously move his head to be able to ogle a passing babe, women have wider peripheral vision.[2] This allows you to fully check out those delicious six-pack abs that are strutting by without ever having to take your eyes off your unsuspecting mate. The drooling, however, might be a tipoff. So dab frequently.

If you're single . . .

Your ovum is pointing you in the direction of men who look like good genetic matchups: They're healthy, strong, and have steady jobs. Or at least they tell you they do.

Sex

A red lace teddy with more peek-a-boo holes than OJ's alibi. A black vinyl corset with Janet Jackson—inspired tearaway cups. Anything Pamela Anderson wears on the Red Carpet. These are just a few of the NC-17 getups that estrogen- and testosterone-fueled high confidence is making you feel utterly sexy and not one bit silly in. Okay, it may be hard to suppress a giggle the first time you try to put on that split crotch thingy. But laughing will be the last thing on his mind when he sees you in it.

Don't cotton to all that Lycra and rubber? Then high confidence will make you feel more comfortable getting completely nude in front of your guy. And if he's like 76 percent of the men out there, he'd prefer it to be with the lights on rather than off.[3] That's because the mere sight of a naked woman is enough to get him fully aroused.[4] Okay, so it's not as if he needs the extra help when it comes to the arousal department. But think of it as foreplay that doesn't muss up your lipstick.

Does worry over your sweetie spotting a butt zit or fat roll have you clapping off while he's clapping on? Well, every moment spent fretting about your appearance is a moment wasted because once you bare your bod all your man sees are hips, breasts, and any postwax pubic hair you have left leading to the pow-zing prize.[5] Blemishes and stretch marks aren't even on his mind. Heck, they're not even in his scope of vision. It's gals who have the detail-oriented eyesight that can spot a freckle 100 tubes of coverup away.[6]

Besides, the more your honey digs you, the more your body looks like sheer unblemished perfection in his eyes. So if you're really anxious about the way you look, all you have to do is pump up the love in your relationship right before climbing into bed. Treat him to a delicious home-made meal, present him with a new video game, or simply tell him how much you care about him. After that, once you drop the robe all he'll see is—well, all he'll still be seeing are hips, breasts, and any postwax pubic hair you have left leading to the pow-zing prize. But they'll all look utterly amazing.

Once you've gotten past the lingerie versus nudity / lights on versus off / boyfriend versus vibrator decisions, high estrogen and testosterone promise to make the time you spend reaching for your O really count. They're giving you the kind of focus that can make you forget all about the dishes that have to be done, the laundry that needs folding, and the boss who keeps leaving irate messages on your answering machine wondering why you're not at work yet. Estrogen has you lubricating with every kiss, touch, and rub. And testosterone is making your orgasms easy to reach and, once reached, feel so all-over intense that you might be inspired to write a sonnet about them. Or at least a haiku.

Money

Splurge alert! If it's for sale, you're buying. And if it's not for sale, you'll be making an offer anyhow. That's buy-till-it's-all-bought-or-go-bankrupt-trying testosterone pushing you to spend as if there's no credit limit. And estrogen is right there by its side quietly reassuring you that you'll be a millionaire any day now so it'll all be okay.

What happened to that left brain analysis that had been trying to keep your spending within limits since Day 6? It's now losing the rock-paper-scissors game to your pumped up, splurge-happy hormones.

Career

High estrogen and testosterone are pumping you full of so much confidence and ambition, you're feeling tempted to go for gigs that you'd recognize as being way out of your league on lower hormone days of the month. For example? Well, say there was a management position opening up. Even if the only supervisory role you've ever had is telling the interns how to make your coffee, you'll be throwing your hat into the ring. Is your boss looking for someone to take over the IT department? Even though you're still searching for the spell check button, you're already picturing how you'll be spending that fat IT paycheck.

Whatever lofty goal you're aiming for, remember that if it's a guy you need to convince, it's best to approach him later in the afternoon when his testosterone decreases, making him less likely to challenge your request. Also limit your proposal to as few words as possible, lower the pitch of your voice and speak slowly. It'll be hard to do even one of these on this chatty, high-pitched, fast talking day. But you'll win him over more easily if you do.

Energy

Relax? What is this thing called "relax"? It's not a word you'll recognize today. But don't worry. It won't even come up while estrogen and testosterone are pumping up your energy to Robert Downey, Jr.-after-a-bender levels. So you won't have to worry too much about it.

Diet

Your sweetie baking his inimitable pineapple upside-down (and all over the kitchen) cake? You're there with two forks and a plate. Your nieces selling, well, you're not sure what, at a bake sale? You buy two. Invited to dinner by a fledgling chef who's teaching herself French cooking? Pas de problème. Even her creative charbroiled snails don't faze you. At least not while you're feeling bolstered by brave testosterone who's pushing you to take tasty risks.

Following Weight Watchers? Trying out the raw foods diet? Inspired by Jared to do the Subway thing? When you're home alone or at work, your left brain makes it easier to stick to your resolutions because you can remember why you made them. But when you're socializing or out on the town, it's a whole 'nother story. It's getting hard not to get swept away in the high estrogen and testosterone excitement and give in to the urge to splurge. Or at least nibble.

Day 12

Not New? Not Fun? Not Worth It!

Mood

Hands up if you remember Day 1. Anyone? Anyone? Here's a refresher: You on the couch in your pilliest PJs, surrounded by a bag of salty pretzels, a pint of chocolate cheesecake ice cream, and the remote, with the hopeful expectations that the phone wouldn't ring, the TV wouldn't give out, and the boy-toy would go on a Motrin and dough-nut run.

Where you are today: You in your slinkiest skirt and struttiest heels out on the town surrounded by three guys you're group dating *Bachelorette*-style, wielding a cell phone with all your best buds conferenced in on walkie-talkie, a half a dozen after-party invites, and the hopeful expectation that practically anything ~~can~~ will happen.

Why the diff? It's all estrogen and testosterone's doing. Over these past eleven days these two hormones have been steadily putting you in the mood to socialize, increasing your energy and blunting the pain caused by squashed toes in high heels. Now optimistic estrogen is reaching the point where it's making you feel invincible. So, no matter what you do, you're pretty sure that you won't land in the ER, morgue, jail, or a segment of *Most Embarrassing Moments Caught on Video*. And impulsive testosterone is reaching the point where you're all about adventure and competitiveness. You not only want to take risks, you want to be the wildest, the wackiest, the one with the most tattoos by the end of the day.

Are your hormones natural or are you taking progesterone-only contraceptives? Then your estrogen and testosterone soar to a level that makes you more willing to do what other people see as clearly dangerous, such as taking on the ten-foot vertical ramp in the skateboard competition, rappelling up the water tower to hang your protest sign, or going canyoning, which, no matter how you slice it, is basically just another way of saying jumping off a really steep, dangerous waterfall and hoping to survive so you can call it a sport. Friends and family urging you to be careful? All you hear is "Yakyakyak. Blahblahblah." Some might say estrogen and testosterone are a bad influence on you. But you know your annual holiday letter would never be as interesting without them.

Taking hormone contraceptives that dole out a constant dose of estrogen? Your estrogen level doesn't soar as high as natural hormones do, so you're less likely to be swept up in the excitement of anything too risky. Oh, you'll still want to get wild. But you're less likely to be okay with the possibility of a body cast just to have a good time.

Slam the brakes on an estrogen stress-out!

Treat yourself to a bowl of ice cream, cookies, cake, or any other kind of yummy comfort food. Turns out, the fat and sugar in these treats stop the production of the adrenal hormones that cause stress!

Less pain, your gain

Bang your knee? You won't even notice. Bump your head? No big deal. Someone pinches you? You'll hardly feel it, but you're not dreaming. It's just high estrogen producing lots of lovely pain-squelching endorphins, making today through Day 14 the lowest pain days of your entire cycle.[1] And that makes it a perfect time to do anything that hurts—such as getting a tooth filling or collagen injections, or breaking in a new pair of heels.

Mind

Since Day 6, you've thought of yourself as a total brainiac. A supergenius with superior verbal, memory, and cognitive skills. So, of course, the idea that high estrogen and testosterone continue to improve these abilities is old news to you. What you may not realize, however, is that today's levels of estrogen and testosterone have you seeing an improvement that even brainiac you may not have anticipated.

Thinking

Where you were recently able to concentrate easily, you can now focus with more intensity than audience members trying to spot themselves on the TV monitor at a *Ricki Lake* taping. While you may have been absorbing new information and making decisions at a rapid rate, you're now learning new facts and calling shots faster than a fading star accepts an invitation to be on *Hollywood Squares*.

Memory

Your memory may have been sharp in recent days, but now everyone better be on their best behavior. You're not forgetting a thing.

Verbal

SAT words that were recently peppering your conversation are now springing out of your mouth with the speed and quantity of coffeecake crumbs.

The side of your brain highlighted today?

Left brain: High estrogen may be pushing you to be daring, but you're still likely to go with what your logical brain says. For instance, estrogen may give you the urge to crash a party, but your logical brain is making sure you pick a party with the most hotties and free booze. And estrogen may be giving you the urge to slip a dude your digits. But your logical brain is making sure you give him the voicemail number in case he turns out to be a jerk. Or worse, a male model.

Day 1 Day 2 Day 3 Day 4 Day 5 Day 6 Day 7

Romance

If you're in a relationship . . .

You love your boy. (No doubt there.) Your relationship is strong; communication is high. (Check. Check.) And any faults he has are so small, you know you could fix them if you really wanted to. (Can loving you too much really be considered an actual fault, anyway?)

And yet, you can't stop staring at the copy repair guy. And the UPS guy. And the water cooler filler guy whom you gazed at as he hoisted two heavy bottles in his big, muscle-bound, perfectly tanned, delicious arms.

So why the roving eye when you love your guy? That's estrogen and testosterone's handiwork. They're like two of Cupid's more impish agents reminding you that love may be a many-splendored thing, but a biological trump card it is not. At least not while they're encouraging you to look around and see if there's an even healthier, more robust sperm donor than the one you've already found to partner with your egg.

If you're single . . .

Single gals on the prowl will be most attracted to men who appear virile, seem as if they can hold down a job, and look strong enough to hoist heavy bottles of water with their big, muscle-bound, perfectly tanned, delicious arms.

Sex

Put your ear to the ground. Hear that rumbling? It's the sound of thousands of men running in your direction. What's luring them? Your pheromones, scentless chemicals your body emits that can attract and arouse a guy more effectively than any $350 bottle of perfume ever could. The closer you get to the day most women traditionally ovulate—Day 14—the more pheromones your body emits. And they're driving the men around you crazy with lust.[2]

Which, of course, they're supposed to do. Think of it as Mother Nature's backup plan. Just in case you ignored all of her pleas to get out there and find a guy, she's turning you into a man magnet by having your body emit the equivalent of a silent dog whistle. Which would explain all of the panting guys sitting outside your door scratching to come in.

Been with your boy toy a few years? Then you may notice his interest in sex has just hit a monthly high. That's because he's getting a double biological whammy from you: He's getting aroused by your increasing pheromones, and since his testosterone has synched up with yours, his testosterone is close to peaking along with yours. This has him practically at the mercy of his near-chronic erection. Happily, your high testosterone is also revving up your own libido. So you'll be racing each other to the bedroom.

Once you give in to testosterone's temptations, it's making sex and masturbation thoroughly fulfilling. Estrogen and testosterone are helping you focus on your body and fantasies. Estrogen is keeping you lubricated and comfortable during thrusting. And testosterone, well, testosterone is giving you what your guy only wishes he could claim responsibility for—easy-to-reach, all-over orgasms that are so extreme, you'll swear they'd qualify as a category in the next X Games.

Money

Looking to fatten your savings account? Then put your hands up and step away from the credit cards. Have a bank account bigger than most European nations? (Or at least giving in to the estrogen- and testosterone-fueled feeling that you do?) Then you'll be tempted to spend on luxury items, such as a tennis bracelet, a Maybach, or your own Gulf Stream jet.

Career

High testosterone is making you ambitious and giving you the impulse to make split-second decisions. So if your boss announces that there's a brand-new position opening for a real go-getter who wants to show off her potential and there is room for growth and, oh, by the way, it's on a deserted island somewhere in the South Pacific, you'll be volunteering yourself in an "oh-no"-second before you realize what you are getting yourself into. Before high testosterone has you packing up your iPod mini and SPF 45 and heading off to an island hut and six months of spear fishing and coconut cracking, take a moment to tap into some of that left brain analysis to double-check that you're making the right decision.

Have any requests you'd like to make to the higher-ups today? For instance, replacing the icky fluorescent lights with more flattering incandescent bulbs, or asking them to rethink that whole "no tongue studs in the workplace" policy? Go for it if your boss is a woman. She'll be able to understand the high-pitched, fast stream of words high estrogen has coming out of your mouth just fine.

If your boss is a guy, however, make your request in "man-speak," the type of communication men use with each other: Limit your use of facial expressions, don't interrupt him, and give a short grunty "hmmm" every now and again while agreeably nodding your head.[3] With so little actual talking going on in men's conversations, it's a wonder they get any communicating done at all. Who knows, maybe there's a secret language encoded in cigars and beer that guys have tried to prevent gals from stumbling across because it reveals just how emotionally sensitive they really are.

Nah. Just go with the grunting.

Energy

You don't wanna just turn the music up. You wanna blow out every woofer and tweeter. You don't wanna just listen to your favorite rock chick. You want to bE tHe RoCk ChICk!!! Ah, energizing estrogen and testosterone—keeping so many stereo stores and karaoke bars in biz.

Diet

A new restaurant. A new recipe. A new kind of frozen pizza. There's a theme here: High testosterone wants you to experiment with food you've never tried before. And high estrogen promises to make it worth your while as it continues to increase your taste buds' sensitivity to flavor.

Counting your saturated fat grams? Cutting out anything with preservatives? On an all-liquid diet? When you're home alone or at work, it's easier to remember to stick to your food restrictions. But if you're at a party or hanging out with friends, high estrogen- and testosterone-fueled enthusiasm have you wanting to let loose, live a little, and try the delicious-looking crab puffs and mini cheese blintzes.

Peak Performance

Day 13

Mood

Once upon a time, millions of years ago, choices in men were limited. There were the hairy, smelly brutes with the clubs. The hairy smelly inventors who could make fire. The hairy, smelly hunters who brought home dinner. And the less hairy and not-nearly-as-smelly interior decorators who showed gals how a beautifully handcrafted clay pot could really dress up a cave.

Since the latter only wanted to be friends, that left even fewer options. So once ovulation approached, a gal needed a gentle push from her hormones to climb into bed with one of these less-than-appealing guys to continue propagating the race.

Today we've got guys who bathe regularly, use deodorant, and have nice cars. Clearly we don't need as much of a push from our hormones to hook up. Too bad our hormones haven't caught on yet.

Since Day 1, estrogen and testosterone have been doing all they could to play matchmaker. Which means

107

that upbeat, optimistic, extroverted mood they were dol-ing out wasn't just a goodwill gift from your biology. It was actually a clever ploy to get you to land a man or to overlook the foibles of the one you have so you'd keep him around at least till today, the day before ovulation, when the possibility for pregnancy is high in women who don't take hormone contraceptives.

It also happens to be when estrogen and testoster-one reach their highest peaks during your entire cycle, whether your hormones are natural or you take hormone contraceptives. What this means for you is that the opti-mism, confidence, extroversion, personal power, derring-do, and fun-loving attitude that have been growing since Day 1 are now peaking, too.

Don't want to have a baby this cycle around? Then use all that hormone-fueled positive thinking and fearless-ness to conceive something else: launch a career, start your own business, go on a road trip, hike the Inca Trail to Machu Picchu, set up a pirate radio station, form a think tank, produce a movie, write a book, record an album, or join the space program.

Nowadays your choices are, indeed, limitless.

Slam the brakes on an estrogen stress-out!

Take a whiff of coconut oil! Scientists have found that breathing in this sweet fragrance lowers your heart rate and reduces stress.[1]

The truth about "safe days"

Sperm—a surprisingly patient bodily secretion—has been known to live up to five days inside a woman.[2] This means unprotected sex you had four days ago could still get you pregnant tomorrow when your egg comes sliding down your fallopian tube. What's more, in an irregular cycle, ovulation can occur days before or after Day 14. Bottom line? Keep the birth control handy all cycle long.

Mind

With estrogen and testosterone peaking, it makes sense that your brain functions peak, too. Ostensibly, this is to help you land a man by the time ovulation comes around. Of course, you can use it for whatever you want . . .

Thinking

Heightened focus keeps you from getting distracted by a killer sale on your way to asking a hunky guy up to your pad; you can use it to concentrate on writing up a comprehensive business plan or coming up with a winning recipe to enter into the annual Pillsbury Bake-Off contest.

Absorbing new facts at a lightning pace enables you to pick up on important—and potentially damning—clues about a potential lover, such as whether he believes that Valentine's Day gifts are merely an evil byproduct of a capitalist regime or he thinks that polygamy is the new monogamy; you can also use this ability to quickly absorb new information by teaching yourself the finer points of electrical engineering or trying out a new cross-stitch.

Making decisions with speed enables you to sift through a party full of eligible bachelors and choose the one you want to take home before the event—and your man-picking opportunity—is over; you can use this ability to make quick decisions about which photos you want to display in your gallery exhibit or what color palette to use during your *Trading Spaces*–inspired redecoration.

Memory

A killer memory enables you to recall which guy at the party had the best pickup line; you can use this skill to remember the formula for pi or to recall which store had those cute shoes you saw in *Marie Claire*.

Verbal

Stellar verbal abilities and major chattiness help you send clear, irrefutable signals to an oblivious guy that you're interested and he should take the bait; you can use these speaking skills to pitch a business investor or perform your one-woman show.

The side of your brain highlighted today?

Left brain: Today's the last day that your logical, practical left brain is influencing you as strongly. Starting tomorrow, when estrogen and testosterone decline and progesterone increases, your brain starts the slow transition to your right brain, which will be complete by Day 20. Till then, if you've got any decisions you want to make that require you to rely more on logic than intuition—like, say, which bank offers the best interest rates or what color eye shadow goes best with your new top—you may want to make them today.

Less Pain, your gain

Your sensitivity to pain reaches a month-long low today. Presumably, this makes it easier to over-look the beard burn your grizzly lover is giving you with his two-day facial growth. You can use it to make the screams from your Brazilian wax a little less eardrum splitting.

The secret way you flirt

From today to Day 15, you're talking in a sing-song voice and using higher and lower notes.[3] Like giggling, eyelash batting, and other uncon-scious flirtatious behaviors, speaking in melodic tones gives you a childlike quality that appeals to a man's primitive urge to protect.[4] Since there are no more saber-toothed tigers roaming around to make your guy feel like the brave hero he yearns to be, make him feel big and strong by asking him to protect you from having to go halfsies on the dinner check.

Romance

If you're in a relationship . . .

Estrogen and testosterone continue to make you feel ga-ga over your guy. He's smart, he's caring, he's got buns of steel. However, you're also feeling an attraction to other men[5]—and estrogen and testosterone are choosing exactly which ones. Want to know who they are? See "If you're single . . . "

If you're single . . .

Estrogen and testosterone are trying to convince you to have sex. But they don't want you to jump in the sack with just anyone, much to the chagrin of hopeful lads everywhere. From Days 13 to 15, feminine-looking guys with less muscle definition than a sea lion, a jawline softer than your Pacific Coast pillow, and who couldn't grow a beard even after a Rogaine facial are out. Manly-looking guys with brawn, stubble, and strong jawlines[6] are so, so in.[7] Some scientists believe this is a hold-over from the early days when cavegals wanted a masculine guy around during ovulation to ensure they were getting the healthiest and strongest genetic matchup for their cave-baby-to-be, but after ovulation they wanted a kinder, more effeminate guy around to help take care of the little cavetyke.[8] *As if.*

Does the superstud you've picked out have a deep voice? That'll draw you in even more since it indicates higher testosterone levels, which translate into a higher probability of conception, which your baby-craving hormones find utterly irresistible. [9]

Is he making his voice even lower as he talks to you? Then not only is he a hottie with a bass voice that'll make you melt, but it's a sure sign that he's into you. If you're into him, the pitch of your own voice will get higher.[10] It's kinda like a horny dueling banjos. But with voices.

So he's got the ripped abs, a chiseled jaw, and a deep voice. Does he get the nod to come into the bedroom? Not just yet. He also has to pass the sniff test. Give him a whiff and in about three seconds you'll know if there's a spark or not. No, it doesn't have to do with determining whether he's wearing top-shelf cologne or a cheap drugstore knockoff. Rather, your nose can detect the state of a man's immune system through the pheromones he's emitting.[11] If his immune system is weaker than yours, no dice. But if your nose detects an immune system that's at least as strong yours, you'll go all-over goofy for him.[12] Biology's reasoning? Complementary immune systems ensure a healthier baby.[13] Not exactly sexy or romantic. But with your knees turning to jelly and your loins virtually on fire, does it really matter?

Okay, so he's manly looking. He's got a bassy voice. And he smells healthy. Is he getting the green light to climb into your bed now? Not quite. There's still one thing that can ax your attraction—if he seems like a lousy potential father.[14] Can't hold a job? Got caught cheating on his last girlfriend? Told you he lost every pet he ever owned? All deal breakers—even if you don't intend to have his little brawny baby. Why? Chalk it up to your biology. It's trying to protect your future investments in case you do decide to have kids down the road with the man you're pursuing tonight.

So he passes all the tests. Your hormones are waving him in. Should you go for it? Well, that depends. If you're the freewheeling type for whom an emotional hangover from sex is as infrequent as a short line at the DMV, by all means, take a walk on the brawny side.

However, if you're the type whose oxytocin immediately bonds you to any guy you have sex with,[15] then before you climb into bed you may want to ask yourself, "Is this the man I imagine my starter marriage being with?" If the answer is anything other than yes, then pull out the list of qualifications you want in a mate that you wrote up on Day 2 to remind yourself of the type of guy you really see yourself regifting duplicate wedding presents with. Otherwise, after oxytocin has you getting all attached to Mr. Muscles after sex, you could mistake today's temporary spark of lust for never-ending true love. And that could have you pulling a Britney and getting a quickie marriage to a guy you'll be serving with divorce papers by Day 16 when the brawn-loving effect wears off.

Sex

In a relationship? Then send your boy toy out of the room. This next part is something you won't want him to read by accident as he reaches over you for the remote: From today till Day 15 peaking estrogen and testosterone are making you most tempted to cheat right now. In fact (is he still out of the room?), you're more likely to have sex with a guy you're keeping on the side than with your own mate.[16]

Oh, you still love him. High estrogen and testosterone are making his every move seem adorable and perfect. So why the itch to roam? Some evolutionary psychologists say premarriage humans developed this biological urge to keep the gene pool diverse, to ensure the healthiest babies, and to give gals a fall-back provider in case her primary mate disappeared. Like, say, when he found out about the other guy.

Sigh. Which influence is a sex-loving but oh-so committed gal to follow? Ultimately, it's your choice. But whether you're in a relationship or single, the guy you pick will be thrilled to hop into bed with you. That's because as you get closer to Day 14, you're emitting more arousal-inducing pheromones than magazines send renewal subscription notices. And this is driving up his libido to gotta-have-you levels. If you decide to have sex with the guy you've been with for years, his testosterone, which has synched up with yours, will also be peaking. That translates into a megadose of do-it-till-you're-sore-or-get-hungry sex.

What about the sex itself? With estrogen and testosterone peaking, it could hardly be better.[17] You're lubricating easily, which makes thrusting more comfortable. You're quick to be aroused and climax is easy to reach. And, once reached, your orgasm is so intense and such an all-over-body experience, you may be inspired to write

115

about it in your blog—and *not* the secret one your friends don't know about either.

Money

Optimistic estrogen and overconfident testosterone are making you feel as if you've got more money than you really do, so you may want to put a limit on your—oh, just go ahead and splurge. Nothing's going to stop you today anyway.

Career

A new chair to replace yours, which has been broken for seven months. The corner office. Real cream instead of that powdered crap. All of this and more are yours for the asking at the office today. Or at least peaking estrogen and testosterone have you confident that they could be. Which is why you may be surprised if any of your requests are turned down.

Did you use the deep voiced, slow-down trick on your guy boss and it still didn't yield the results you wanted? Or worse—did someone else get what he or she asked for while you didn't? High estrogen and testosterone don't believe in keeping emotions under wraps. So you'll likely feel the impulse to express your disappointment. Perhaps by sending an e-mail throughout the office filled with really angry emoticons such as >>:- (. Or by stabbing your stress ball with the spork from your midday salad. Just be sure no tattletale coworkers are around to capture it on their camera phone and submit it to the company newsletter. Spork stabbing is not a pretty look on you.

Energy

With estrogen and testosterone at their peak, energy and endurance are as high as they're going to get this cycle. So today's the day to do anything that requires maximum drive and stamina—say, mountain biking the advanced trail, wallpapering the entire house, or cleaning out your black hole of a purse.

Diet

When estrogen peaks, so do your taste buds' sensitivity to flavor. When testosterone peaks, so does your sense of adventure for trying new foods. Sensitive to flavor? Willing to try new foods? This is a recipe for a potluck if there ever was one.

On a diet? The bad news is that high estrogen still makes it more difficult to resist splurging at a party or when hanging with the buds. The good news? You're eating 12 percent less than you will be tomorrow through Day 28.

Pap smear alert!

Day 13 is the best day to have a Pap smear to detect cervical cancer. That's because around ovulation, cervical mucus is thinnest. And this yields the best sampling of cells, which increases the odds of discovering cancer in its earliest, most treatable state.[18]

Will you be ovulating tomorrow?

To find out, use a "saliva ovulation tester," a reusable lipstick-shaped minimicroscope that determines the level of estrogen in your body by measuring the amount of salt in your saliva. When estrogen peaks, so does the salt in your saliva. And that indicates that it's one day before ovulation. The following day will be the day you ovulate. You can purchase a reusable saliva ovulation tester in drugstores or online for $20 to $60.

Turning Point

Cycle Check: Is Today Your Day 14?

Have a 28-day cycle? Take 28-day hormone contraceptives?

Then today is your Day 14. So read Day 14 today.

Don't have a 28-day cycle and have natural hormones?

Whether or not you read Day 14 today depends on one little thing—it's about the size of the period at the end of this sentence, in fact—your egg. In "How to Use This Book," you learned how to tell when your egg has been released from your ovary, which signals that you're ovulating. If you followed that advice, then here's how it breaks down:

- If you're ovulating today: Read Day 14 today. You're right on schedule with the typical 28-day cycle.
- If you ovulated before Day 14: Read Day 14 today. Based on the advice from "How to Use This Book," you

119

probably already jumped ahead from whatever day you ovulated. Your menstrual cycle is likely shorter than the average 28-day cycle. If your cycle is consistent, in about three months you'll know when your usual Day 14 falls. You'll also get a feel for how much faster you go through the first half of your cycle than a typical 28-dayer. If it's not consistent, continue to track your ovulation.

- If you haven't ovulated yet: Don't read Day 14 till ovulation occurs. For now, reread Day 13. When you ovulate move on to Day 14. Your menstrual cycle is probably longer than the typical 28-day cycle. If your cycle is consistent, in about three months you'll know when your usual Day 14 falls. You'll also get a feel for how much more slowly you go through the first half of your menstrual cycle than a typical 28-dayer. If it's not consistent, continue to track your ovulation.

Take Seasonale, the 91-day pill?

Day 14 comes 38 days after the first day of your period. That's because during your cycle, you read Days 1 to 6 one day each and each subsequent chapter four days each.

And what about Days 15 to 28?

The first half of your menstrual cycle is the only part that varies in length. The second half is usually a consistent 14 days.[1] So Day 15 to Day 28 should match up just right with rest of your cycle.

Didn't track ovulation?

Then you can simply match up your mood characteristics with each day's description to put yourself back on track.

Pre-PMS Alert!

Here's something you may have suspected, but probably were never told about in health class—pre-premenstrual syndrome.[2] Starting today and lasting till Day 18, pre-PMS is a lot like the usual PMS, but it's shorter and less intense. Kinda like the bunny hill. Or Nicky Hilton.

The reason pre-PMS and PMS are so similar is that both are caused by the same thing: declining hormones. In pre-PMS, estrogen and testosterone are decreasing. In PMS, estrogen and testosterone are joined by progesterone in the downward slide.[3]

What makes decreasing hormones such a bummer? Just like anything else that's addictive—caffeine, cigarettes, Krispy Kreme doughnuts—your body gets hooked. So once these hormones decline, your body goes through withdrawal.[4] It's these withdrawal symptoms that people are really referring to when they talk about PMS.

If you've ever wondered why one gal's PMS feels as bland as an Ashlee Simpson video while another gal feels as if she's been shoved and trampled by J-Lo's entourage, a lot of it depends on your sensitivity to hormones. If you're not sensitive to hormones, then withdrawal symptoms will be mild and pop up only occasionally. If you're sensitive to hormones, then withdrawal symptoms will be intense and frequent.[5]

Which hormone contraceptive you take also plays a role in how you experience pre-PMS and PMS. If yours contains progesterone only, then your estrogen and testosterone levels are similar to a woman with natural hormones. That means both hormones plunge today, so you're feeling the full force of pre-PMS.

If your hormone contraceptives contain estrogen, however, then your estrogen and testosterone don't reach the same highs or lows that other women do. But this doesn't mean you escape pre-PMS altogether. Turns out, many women report that they still experience cyclical changes similar to their natural menstrual cycle. Some researchers believe it's because your body's other hormones and brain chemicals have cyclical fluctuations. Other researchers speculate that a woman's own natural hormones may be breaking through and causing cycle fluctuations. Whatever the reason, you'll likely experience a milder version of pre-PMS.

Want to know which hormone causes which symptom? Of course you do. How else will you know which one to curse out when you feel a withdrawal symptom coming on?

Testosterone withdrawal diminishes self-confidence.[6] It makes you feel like, even after going over the same task forty-eight times, a Spice Girl could have done a better job. It also makes risky adventures seem too unsafe to engage in and has you feeling pretty sure that anyone who does something as crazy as bungee jumping, skydiving, or canyoneering is just asking for a full body cast.

Estrogen withdrawal makes you experience bouts of nervousness, anxiety, teariness, and the blues—usually not related to any specific event that's happening around you.[7] They just show up unannounced. Kinda like that stoner kid in your dorm who could hear a pizza being delivered from two floors away.

Estrogen withdrawal is also the cause of another notorious hallmark of pre-PMS and PMS: the temper flare. Caused by a surge of noradrenaline, this brain chemical can actually affect you in two ways: It can give you that heart-pounding, flash-of-anger feeling you get when a car suddenly veers in front of you and you let loose with a string of swear words that rivals a transcript from a Colin Farrell interview. Or it can give you that exuberant, joyful feeling you get when all the numbers on your lottery ticket come up. Or your boyfriend does the dishes.

You probably won't mind it when noradrenaline makes you happy. But that noradrenaline temper flare, well, let's just say throwable objects tremble in its presence.

Luckily, noradrenaline temper flares aren't invincible. There is one brain chemical that can squash noradrenaline into submission—serotonin, a substance that helps stabilize mood and elevate good feelings.

What gives serotonin this awesome power? Well, it's like this: Serotonin and noradrenaline are like two school kids on a seesaw. One goes up, the other goes down. But both can't be up at the same time.[8] From Day 1 to Day 13, serotonin was usually always the one that was up because elevated levels of estrogen kept it high. But now that estrogen is decreasing, serotonin's been decreasing. And that's been giving noradrenaline a chance to be on the upside of that seesaw.

If you boosted good-guy serotonin so it went back up, it would push down mean ol' noradrenaline. And that would keep your mood stable and convince your boyfriend to come out of hiding.

Now if there was only a way to boost serotonin . . . Good news—there is. In fact, there are lots of ways. That's because serotonin rises whenever you do something fun or indulgent (such as shopping or getting a facial) or whenever you do something good for your body (such as exercise, massage, or—stock up on your batteries now—masturbation).[9]

Even better news: Whether you have mild or severe withdrawal symptoms, these anxiety spells, blue moods, and noradrenaline temper flares aren't a constant plague throughout your day. They merely pop up every now and then to interrupt your regularly scheduled mood.

Sure-fire serotonin booster

Eat a cookie, scarf some fudge, nibble some cake, or indulge in any other sweet treats. Research shows that sugar increases serotonin levels!

Mood

Day 14 ushers in the second half of your cycle and marks the descent of estrogen and testosterone and the rise of progesterone. The first thing you'll notice about this second phase is that feelings of optimism begin to wane and you're less likely to gloss over problems and issues.[10] Oh, it's not like at the stroke of midnight your boyfriend suddenly turns from quaintly unkempt to disgusting slob. And your job doesn't immediately transform from total dream gig to the soul-sucking thing you do for a paycheck. But over the next few days, you will notice that the rosy hue through which you've viewed life since Day 1 is wearing off.

As estrogen and testosterone decrease, they're also taking away all that superconfidence you had in your appearance and talents and replacing it with seeds of self-doubt.[11] What's more, your interest in daring stunts and exotic locales is slowly being replaced by a desire to feel comforted and safe.[12]

Progesterone, a hormone known for its sedative qualities, dominates for the next two weeks. So you'll enjoy a sense of soothing calm that makes you feel as though you can get through any high stakes situation with nary a stomach churn or sweat bead rolling over you.[13]

If you're sensitive to hormones, then progesterone may also usher in bouts of the blues, feelings of being overwhelmed or even depression.[14] Not a day at the spa to be sure, but this definitely qualifies as a free pass to treat yourself like a queen and indulge in all the spending sprees, truffle munchies, and blog rants that you can fit in till your mood perks up again on Day 1, when progesterone bottoms out and estrogen and testosterone begin their steady, mood-lifting rise again.

Nesting alert!

Day 14 through Day 28 you'll feel the urge to vacuum the rug, straighten the pictures, fluff the couch cushions, and go to Pier 1 to charge $200 in home accents. That's progesterone's influence. It's giving you the urge to beautify your home and make it more comfy-cozy. This is an ancient nesting instinct that had gals dolling up the cave with bison-skin throw rugs and straw accent baskets. Today, it keeps you knee-deep in aromatherapy candles and twig balls.

Mind

Estrogen and testosterone decline today, which signals the declining of your brain skills and the start of the transition from your left brain to your right brain. However, since both hormones are still relatively high, the difference is less of a clap-on/clap-off and more like a Japanese tea ceremony— you really have to appreciate it for its subtlety.

Thinking

Quick—which would you prefer: killer concentration, the ability to absorb new information instantly, or lightning-speed decision making? Luckily, it doesn't matter which you choose, since all your brain skills are still sharp even as your hormones turn tail. But now you know which one you woulda picked. And that's useful for, well, nothing really. Good thing you're still feeling too smart to care.

Memory
Your recall may not be improving anymore, but you've still got the kind of memory that makes you wonder how you could ever forget where you put your keys, the name of the intern who always says hi to you, and all 138 tasks on your to-do list.

Verbal
Appearances can be deceiving. A dandelion looks like a flower. It's actually a weed. Mike Tyson looks like a bass. Really, he's a soprano. You *look* as if you don't have much to say. Really you're a verbal Venus flytrap should anyone get too close. The reason? As talkative estrogen and testosterone fall and quieting progesterone rises, your urge to chat decreases. But once you do start to talk, you're firing multisyllabic arrows in the direction of any-one who dares try to go toe-to-toe, slicing up others' arguments with the skill of a medical examiner performing an autopsy, and presenting your case more persuasively than a prosecutor waving DNA evidence.

The side of your brain highlighted today?
Left brain: While there may not seem to be much change in brain skills on the first day estrogen and testosterone decline, this decreasing trend does signal the beginning of the transition from your logical and analyzing left brain to the creative and imaginative right.[15] The shift

Day 1 Day 2 Day 3 Day 4 Day 5 Day 6 Day 7

won't be complete till Day 20, but over the next few days you might notice that while doing left brain tasks—such as measuring, organizing, editing, researching, or budgeting—you may get struck with flashes of creative ingenuity. For instance, while doing your budget, you may come up with an inventive idea that can save you money, say, not buying any more books on how to save money.

Be a math whiz all cycle long!

Declining estrogen and testosterone are decreasing the confidence you have in your appearance and that's bringing down your math skills. Why? Turns out, a woman's self-assessment of her appearance is tied to her perception of her math ability. So the better you think you look, the better you'll actually do; the worse you think you look, the worse you'll do.[16] Happily, simply wearing something flattering and comfortable can help bump your math abilities right back up.[17]

Less pain, your gain

Getting your eyebrows waxed? Letting your friend practice acupuncture on you? Breaking in a new underwire bra? Estrogen may be on the decline but it's still high enough to keep your pain threshold at near-peak levels, which makes the usual ouch inducers a little less agonizing.

Romance

If you're in a relationship . . .

Estrogen and testosterone may be on the decline but they're still at relatively high levels. So if you're attached, while they no longer have you overlooking absolutely all of your boy-toy's foibles, most of them still remain below the radar. And while they may no longer have you feeling as though you and your man are on such a similar wavelength that you can each anticipate what the other is about to say even when you're not in the same room, you can still finish most of each other's sentences when you're just a few feet apart.

However, no matter how faultless he seems or how close your relationship feels, your hormones still have you peeking around at all the other lads in a last ditch effort to find the strongest and healthiest genetic matchup. You know, just in case your guy isn't it.

If you're single . . .

The kind of men who are most likely to catch your attention today are the burly, square-jawed, thick-eyebrowed type. You know, a total Buzz Lightyear. He'll be even more attractive if he's got a deep voice, passes the "sniff" test that reveals whether his immune system is strong, and doesn't come off as potential deadbeat daddy material.

Sex

The good news for you: Even though estrogen and testosterone begin to dip, they're still at relatively high levels, so you continue to have a high libido. Plus, your body is emitting lots of man-magnet pheromones, which only increase your guy's devotion to you.

The not-so-good news for him: Even though he's paying more attention to you, you're more likely to be unfaithful today. Between your boy toy's tears, console him by explaining that it's not because you don't love him anymore. Rather, around this time of month your hormones push you toward more masculine-looking, muscle-bound guys in order to secure the strongest and healthiest genes for your egg.

Then again, you might be better off keeping that whole masculine-looking, muscle-bound bit to yourself and blaming your wandering eye on his inability to throw his dirty socks in the hamper. This strategy won't curb your urge to cheat, but it might just put a stop to your ever having to touch a stinky piece of cloth that's been soaking up your guy's foot sweat all day long.

Whoever you decide to bring into bed, or whether you choose to go it alone, near-peak estrogen and testosterone make sex and masturbation simply astounding. Estrogen has you lubricating with every touch, which makes thrusting more comfortable. And testosterone is getting you easily aroused, making you fast to climax, and turning your orgasm into such a thrilling event, you just might cancel your whitewater rafting trip and go for another round of bedroom fun instead.

Money

When estrogen and testosterone plunge, that secure millions-in-the-bank feeling goes right along with them. Bills you so cavalierly put aside during rising hormone days begin to worry you. And you begin to become concerned that you'll never be able to reach future financial goals—such as buying a house, touring Europe, or affording a new pair of Manolo Blahniks by the time the next spring collection comes out.

But all this doesn't mean you're done spending just yet. That's because, even though they're on the downslide, right now these two hormones are still at relatively high—and impulse-buying—levels. So if you've got your eye on something big, you may want to sneak it in while your hormones are still looking the other way.

"Awww" alert!

From today to Day 28 you're more susceptible to buying anything that uses a rosy-cheeked tyke or fuzzy-faced baby animal to sell it. That's progesterone's fault. It's a hormone that makes women become instantly emotional at the mere sight of babies of any species, plus anything else that >>

>> might resemble a stubby, doe-eyed baby shape, including teddy bears, Winnie the Pooh cartoons, and chubbily adorable comic actor Jack Black.[18] Nature intended this reaction to spur lactation in new moms and make all women want to nurture anything that looks all cuddewy wuddewy. However, once marketing execs learned about progesterone's effects, they discovered they could harness it to get you to buy anything from carrot peelers to vacation property just by filling the ads with infants and puppies.[19]

Career

Put your power suit back in the closet. Close the Machiavelli e-book you've been reading on your PDA. Take the life coach off retainer. You won't feel like using these career-propelling tools again till the beginning of your next menstrual cycle. That's because, with testosterone on the decline, that urgent ambition to rise to the top begins to wane. Oh, it's not gone completely. The corner office and your own parking space still sound pretty sweet. But you won't feel like taking out your coworkers Karate Kid–style to get them. In fact, every now and again decreasing testosterone has you questioning just how secure you feel at your job and wondering if this is even the place you want to take over in ~~five years~~ ~~three years~~ ~~two years~~ by your next menstrual cycle. But rest assured, by Day 1 you'll be slashing your Mont Blanc through the office like a swashbuckling pirate once again.

Till then, it's your coworkers who really benefit from your descending testosterone. As your competitive spirit declines, you become more open to collaborating with others. And you've got lots to bring to the table. Since you're still in your left brain phase, your analyzing skills are sharp. And though beginning to decline from their Superwoman phase, you're still near the high end of your verbal, memory, and cognitive cycles. All this makes you an excellent addition to any team that needs someone to pore over reports, produce spreadsheets, edit proposals, or do any other task where dotting the i's and crossing the t's translates into big $$$.

Energy

No one's naming names, but someone's energy and endurance begin to decrease today. Part of the reason for this slow-down is that estrogen and testosterone are declining. When that happens, they take all the exuberant vigor and stamina they gave you right along with them.[20]

But an even bigger reason for your energy decline is progesterone. If there's one thing you should know about this hormone it's that it has a calming influence. In fact, it's been shown to be eight times more powerful than a common barbiturate.[21] And *way* more powerful than your Sleepytime herbal tea.

Diet

From Days 1 to 13, estrogen and testosterone were holding the menu. Now it's progesterone's turn to order. And what progesterone has you craving are familiar foods you love, especially sweets, salts, carbs, and fats.[22]

On a diet? There's good news: If you don't start to indulge, it's easier to stave off junk food cravings for the entire two progesterone-dominated weeks.[23] What's more, if you do get hit with a craving you think you simply can't resist, going for a simple ten-minute walk will step it down from that gotta-eat-it-or-die-trying level.[24]

But regardless of whether you choose healthy, nutritious foods or set up camp in the bakery aisle, you're eating 12 percent more from today through Day 28.[25] That's because progesterone is making your blood sugar more sensitive, which means you're feeling hungry every three or four hours instead of every five to six.[26] If you don't heed your tummy's urge to nosh, it can make you irritable, dizzy, or light-headed, and give you a headache. Graze all day and you'll keep the food crankies away.[27]

One other thing: It's time to include more fiber in your diet. That's because progesterone is slowing down your digestive tract, which can make you constipated.[28] While mildly annoying because of the bloat and heaviness, constipation can also cause headaches and hemorrhoids, and contribute to those dastardly yeast infections which are surely the work of some misogynist devil.[29] Luckily, fiber doesn't have to be as drab tasting as it sounds. In fact, it can be as easy as switching from Ritz crackers to Triscuits, Cinnamon Toast Crunch to Frosted Mini-Wheats and chocolate chip cookies to oatmeal raisin. Now you don't have to feel guilty about asking your friend to pass the bag of Pepperidge Farms! They're medicinal!

Health

The sudden downturn in estrogen and testosterone does more than disrupt a good mood. It can spark body pain, too:

- Migraine alert: The sudden drop in estrogen makes today through Day 17 a red alert time for migraine sufferers.[30]
- Sports injury alert: Today women are close to three times as likely to sustain a tear of the anterior cruciate ligament on the inside of the knee that connects the thigh bone with the shin bone. It's a common injury affecting athletes, particularly those who play sports that involve a lot of running, jumping, twisting, and turning, such as aerobics, soccer, softball, and volleyball.[31]
- One in four women who ovulate will feel a pain by their ovary. Called Mittelschmerz (meaning "middle pain"), it's caused by the rupture of an egg from the ovary. The sensation ranges from mild, brief twinges to severe, lingering pain, sometimes accompanied by slight bleeding.[32]

The Dark Side of the Moon

Mood

The first half of your menstrual cycle was a wild ride while it lasted. If you played your cards right, estrogen and testosterone had you Frenching Iggy Pop in the bathroom at CBGBs, drinking far too many Guinness pints at an Irvine Welsh reading, and taking your company public. Or, if you're less NYC and more LA, your hormones had you doing a dance-off with Justin Timberlake at Hollywood's Sunset Room, drinking far too many apple martinis at a celeb-studded movie premiere, and expanding your company to include a line of jewelry, cosmetics, and perfume.

Didn't get the chance to indulge in such high-flying, daring adventures this time around? You probably still managed to give in to the temptation to be bold in other ways, perhaps by bravely trying a new pizza topping, fearlessly making an MP3 mix for the guy you're crushing on, or shamelessly scarfing your roommate's last Häagen-Dazs ice cream bar and blaming it on the dog.

So what happens now? Let's just say that the second half of your menstrual cycle is a little less *Real World* and a lot more *Starting Over*. As estrogen and testosterone decline, you become more introspective than extroverted, you face issues with a more realistic than hopeful view, you begin to second-guess yourself as the super self-assuredness you had slowly fades, and the fearless adventurer in you makes way for a gal who prefers the comfort and predictability of home.

As always with declining estrogen and testosterone, you also continue to experience pre-PMS withdrawal symptoms, such as bouts of nervousness, anxiety, the blues, insecurity, and noradrenaline temper flares. Depending on your hormone sensitivity and which hormone contraceptive you take, these symptoms will be as gentle and rare as a joke made by an NPR talk show host or as jarring and frequent as porn spam in your e-mail inbox.

Sure-fire serotonin booster

Open the curtains and let in more light. Or go for a daytime stroll. Studies show that sunlight boosts your body's level of vitamin D, which increases serotonin!

Mind

Today you begin the transformation from your Superwoman brain skills phase to your ordinary girl-without-superpowers phase. Sound like bad news? Not so. First of all, even when you reach the lowest point on your verbal, memory, and cognitive scales—which doesn't happen till Day 28—it's still not as if it's a total bobble-head situation. You're simply returning to the normal level of brain skills that most every guy and low hormone gal has. That Superwoman phase was just giving you an extra advantage.

Thinking

While on their way down, your powers of concentration, ability to grasp new info, and decision-making skills are still relatively high. So if you procrastinated so long you missed the past few Superwoman days, you get a free pass today.

Memory

Like your thinking skills, your memory is still pretty sharp today. But starting tomorrow, that intern goes back to being called "Hey you."

Verbal

This is the one brain skill where you'll notice a decline. That's because progesterone interferes with verbal ability.[1] Which means you may catch yourself stumbling over words that came flowing effortlessly out of your mouth just a day or two ago, or perhaps find yourself inexplicably pausing before answering a question or in the middle of a sentence.[2] These first few verbal stumbles don't stop you from continuing to dominate the conversation, however. Even though you're initiating slightly fewer chats and bringing up a tad fewer topics of your own as quieting progesterone rises and estrogen and testosterone fall, once you do get started, you've still got lots to say. So if Ed from accounting was planning to interrupt with his story about refinishing his boat, he'll have to wait till a lower estrogen and testosterone day.

The side of your brain highlighted today?

Left brain to right brain: As estrogen and testosterone continue to descend and progesterone takes center stage, your right brain takes over and a whole new set of useful brain tools comes into play—like creativity, brainstorming, and problem-solving skills. They don't reach full force till Day 20, though you will see sparks of what's in store during the next few days.

Romance

If you're in a relationship . . .

Your guy's secret wish? That your menstrual cycle lasted only from Days 1 to 13. Can you really blame him though? That was when rising estrogen and testosterone had you blind to virtually all his faults. Even after he crashed your car and lost your cat, it still felt as if he could do no wrong.

No such luck on Days 14 through 28. Now he's got to be on his best behavior as declining estrogen and testosterone dull that optimistic glow and help you see his faults in a whole new, realistic light.

139

If your mate plays it smart, today he'll lay low and shower you with compliments and gifts. *Many* gifts. That's because this is the final day that your hormones are pushing you to check out other lads who might be stronger and healthier genetic matchups for your ovum. And the last thing your mate wants to do is mess up and push you into the understanding—and oh-so muscular—arms of another guy.

If you're single . . .

Your hormones continue to keep you on the hunt for a macho sperm—and it doesn't care who the macho sperm belongs to. Is his apartment decorated with bikini babe posters? His only mode of transportation a scooter—and it's not even electric? Does he admit to owning the entire Frat Rock collection? Three strikes on most days of the month for sure. But on Day 15, the final day of ovulation in a typical fertile cycle, if he's got a strong jaw, a deep voice, and a healthy scent, your hormones will have you overlooking even these transgressions, which would otherwise have spelled game over for Mr. Stud.

Sex

Cupid's conundrum: Your libido remains high and you continue to emit loads of lad-attracting pheromones that have your guy just waiting for the "go" signal. The problem is that feisty pre-PMS noradrenaline, a chemical that bursts on the scene whenever irritation is high, is waiting around the corner threatening to preempt your good time at the first sign that your mate might do something stupid to provoke it. And let's face it, now that decreasing estrogen and testosterone are taking the everything-he-does-is-A-OK lens off the camera through which you're viewing life, the odds of him saying something stupid have increased exponentially.

There is, of course, only one solution: Squeeze in sex in the morning before your guy has a chance to say or do something irritating that summons up lust-busting noradrenaline.

Are you too late? Did he already use up all your Bioré pore strips to make a papier-mâché piñata or tell you he accidentally dropped your toothbrush in the toilet . . . yesterday? Then you may be tempted to give in to the urge to climb into another man's bed. Not simply because it gives you another shot at jumping a guy before he screws it all up by sparking another noradrenaline burst. But also because your hormones continue to encourage you to take another dip into the gene pool just to make sure there isn't a lad who's got healthier and stronger sperm for your egg. That you also get another shot at sex before a guy can say something to mess it up just happens to be an added bonus.

Regardless of who you decide to bring to bed, or if you choose to head for the vibrator for a little DIY action, you definitely don't want to miss out on the total mind-blowing orgasms that still relatively high testosterone is practically handing you on a silver platter today.

Money

Spending seemed so easy and fun from Day 1 to 13. But as estrogen and testosterone plunge, so does the rosy sheen that kept you protected from the truth about your dwindling bank balance. And that's having you—gasp!—hesitate when it comes to doling it out now.

But your favorite stores shouldn't get their bankruptcy papers ready just yet. While estrogen and testosterone are falling, they're still at relatively high levels. So you may feel a pang of worry over big purchases, but you'll likely have little problem giving in to smaller testosterone-fueled impulse buys.

Career

Decreasing estrogen and testosterone continue to ramp down the inner take-over titan in you. And that has you less inclined to want to run the show and more likely to team up and pool resources.

Do skeptical coworkers want to know why you suddenly want to join forces after spending Days 1 through 13 trying to bump them out of the way on your rise to the top? You can tell them that you've grown, you're wiser, and you're ready to hear to what they have to contribute. (Truth? Declining estrogen and testosterone are making you a tad quieter and more interested in listening than leading the conversation.) You can tell them you've got lots to offer. (Without a doubt. Your cognitive, memory, and verbal skills may be on the decline, but you're not even close to being down for the count.) And you can tell them it's because you enjoy their company. (Until someone tries to eat the last chocolate croissant. Then you may be tempted to drop a noradrenaline bomb on their pastry-stealing ass.)

Energy

Decreasing estrogen and testosterone are lowering your energy level and progesterone is making you feel sedate. However, you still have enough vitality and endurance to make it through a full day of band rehearsals and a gig at night. You just might not feel like swinging your guitar over your head and smashing it onstage. Instead you might just rebelliously throw a pick out at the audience. Hey, it's still pretty daring—it could put an eye out.

Fat-burning alert!

Exercise feels easier to do and burns up to 30 percent more fat today through Day 26! Researchers say it's because the estrogen and progesterone combo during this phase promotes the use of body fat as energy.[3] But who cares why when it translates into 30 percent less guilt per cookie!

Diet

Progesterone has you hankering for familiar treats and comfort foods from childhood—such as pizza, peanut butter and jelly, SpaghettiOs, cookies, ice cream, and Froot Loops. And if you've already given in to the cravings for sweets, salts, carbs, and fats, then you're craving them even more.

Regardless of whether you give in to temptations or stick with the nutritious stuff, you'll still be getting hungry every three to four hours. That's because progesterone continues to make your blood sugar sensitive. Ignore the hunger pangs and you can become irritable, dizzy, and lightheaded, and get a headache. Eat small meals all day long and it will help keep your mood level and your body feeling just right.

Since progesterone slows down digestion, which can bring constipation and ensuing headaches, hemorrhoids, and yeast infections, continue to add fiber to your diet. You can opt for the chalky powders you add to drinks and hope to swill it before you taste it. Or you can simply eat high-fiber foods, such as salad, beans, and brown rice.

Leggo My Eggo

Mood

Today is the day your hormones believe the opportunity to get pregnant this time around has officially ended. (However, pregnancy can still happen anyway, so keep those condoms handy!) As a result, estrogen and testosterone are no longer pushing you to land a man. And an amazing thing happens: You're hanging up the micromini and reaching for your comfiest Old Navy sweats, trading in the high heels for a cozy pair of slippers, and using the time you'd spend cruising oxygen bars and techie conventions to catch up on your *Entertainment Weekly*s and learn conversational French.

The theme here? The rest of your menstrual cycle is all about you. Reviewing your big issues, reassessing your goals, and getting back in touch with the little things you love to do, such as knitting, baking, hiking, reading. You know, all the activities you were too busy to get to during the first half of your menstrual cycle, when you were hunting down stud-filled parties.

Depending on your hormone sensitivity and which kind of hormone contraceptive you use, you continue to experience either mild or intense side effects of estrogen and testosterone withdrawal—like bouts of agitation, melancholy, self-doubt, or insecurity.

In between pre-PMS symptoms, lower levels of estrogen and testosterone make you thoughtful and introspective. And tranquilizing progesterone is making you feel calm and serene. If you happen to be sensitive to hormones, you may find progesterone is bringing on a bit of the blues.

Whatever your hormone sensitivity, progesterone is nudging you into a nurturing phase.[1] This means you're feeling the urge to cook more (or at least be the one to call for takeout), brew a cup of raspberry tea for your mate (don't tell him it came from your PMS herbal tea collection till after he says he loves it), and straighten your home to make it more comfortable for the cocooning days ahead (oh, and will there be cocooning).

Sure-fire serotonin booster

Burn a vanilla-scented candle, dab on vanilla essential oil, or simply take a whiff of vanilla extract. Research shows that simply breathing in the scent of vanilla increases serotonin!

Mind

Just as your verbal skills began to do yesterday, today your memory and cognitive skills begin to slide toward the low end of their cycles.[2]

Thinking

Brain skills are slipping from their superhigh state of, well, yesterday. But the difference is only a smidge. For instance, you may notice your mind wandering once or twice at times when you're trying to concentrate on tasks—such as doing an Excel spreadsheet or counting how many times your roommate says "dude" in a single sentence. If you're whipping up a new paella recipe or putting together a bookcase, you might need to read the directions more than once. And decisions you'd usually make in an instant—such as whether to guilt out a tele-marketer by telling him he interrupted you in the middle of putting out a kitchen fire or to simply tell him to go to hell and hang up—take a moment longer to consider.

Memory

While your memory is still sharp enough to recall most names, dates, and facts, you might find one or two details slipping through the cracks.

Verbal

Progesterone continues yesterday's trend of placing a few hesitations in your speech and putting words that you've used in the past three days right at the tip of your tongue but not quite into your conversation. While these verbal stumbles don't slow you down, decreasing estrogen and testosterone are, since the lower they go, the less interested you become in having an all-out chatfest.

The side of your brain highlighted today?

Left brain to right brain: You move one step further from your logical left brain and one step closer to your creative right brain. During this transition, you're getting the best of both sides—practicality with occasional bursts of imagination and intuition. Which means if you've got a decision to make, you might feel the urge to hit Google to do research and then turn to your tarot cards for a second opinion.

Romance

If you're in a relationship . . .

Here's a bit of welcome news for your guy: Your hormones are no longer pushing you to flirt with every lad who crosses your path. Your focus is now squarely on your mate.

Here's some not-so-welcome news for your guy: Your newly focused attention on your mate comes at the same time fault-hiding estrogen and testosterone take a tumble. This alignment has you seeing all his flaws in an oh-no-you-did-not, realistic light.

If you're single . . .

Did you bring home a square-jawed, deep-voiced, macho hunk these past three days? Then when the first morning rays of sunlight poke you in the eyes and give you a good look at the scruffy mound of unwashed muscles lying next to you, your involuntary gasp will be the signal that your high fertility phase—and the He-Man-loving party—is, indeed, over. That's because today you return to being attracted to gentler, more feminine-looking guys who don't leave you with beard burn and who'll sit and watch *Ellen* with you without complaining.

If sex hasn't already produced enough bond-to-you-like-glue oxytocin to make you feel attached to him, then there's still time to usher your midcycle muscleman out the door and tell him he's welcome to try his luck again in twenty-six days.

If you're already hooked on Mr. Wrong On More Days Than He's Right, then run out now and get a Mach3 Turbo razor, a bottle of Vera Wang cologne, and Kiehl's alcohol-free herbal toner for men and make him use all three. Yes, your rough-and-tumble honey will complain. That is, till you patiently explain that bringing out his softer side gives him a fighting chance to last with you the rest of the month. What? You thought metrosexuals were born that way?

$\int e^x$

Testosterone is decreasing to a point where it's putting a slight damper on your sex drive, and progesterone is "plugging up" testosterone receptors in your brain, so you feel even less of the libido-boosting hormone. This doesn't mean you've completely lost interest in sex overnight. You won't be pulling out the chastity belt and letting the hair grow on your legs just yet. For now, you'll merely notice that all things sexual start to get a tad less intense. For instance, instead of steamy thoughts popping into your head with every blink, they're waiting till every other blink. Instead of having orgasms in seconds, it's taking a couple of minutes longer. And rather than a ten-toe curler, your orgasm is more like an eight or a nine.

Here's one more reason you may be less inclined to leap into the sack with a guy: You don't have the confidence about your body that you did during the first half of your cycle. That's because during the second half, decreasing estrogen and testosterone have you feeling self-doubt about your appearance and fretting over every line, bump, and wrinkle that you didn't give a second thought to on high estrogen and testosterone days. To add snack cake to injury, rising progesterone is making you hungrier more often, intensifying your cravings, and sending you on a comfort food bender, which has you feeling like a gazillion pounds.

Okay, truth? Your weight is less of an issue with men than you think. Surveys consistently show that guys prefer plump over skinny.[3] And it's not ice cream companies commissioning these surveys either. Lads simply have a biological preference for women with curves.[4] In fact, researchers have even pinpointed the exact body curve that turns men on the most: a waist measurement that's between 67 percent and 80 percent of that of your hips.[5] It's this hip-to-waist ratio that indicates high fertility and a strong immune system, which a guy's brain is wired to recognize.[6]

But luring men isn't the only reason progesterone increases cravings and encourages you to pack on the pounds. Storing fat is your body's way of preparing for when it's time to nurse. During lactation, it's the fat from your hips and thighs that's accessed for the milk supply.[7]

What's more, once you reach menopause, having a few extra pounds makes the transition easier. The reason? Estrogen is stored in fat cells. So women who reach menopause and stop producing estrogen can rely on the estrogen in their fat to make menopause symptoms less intense.[8]

Bottom line: Progesterone is no dummy. It wants you to eat that cookie for your own good. So why fight it? It's so much yummier to give in.

Money

What will you feel like doing with your money now that testosterone has decreased enough to take away all that millions-in-the-bank confidence and estrogen has decreased enough to take away all that "Bill collectors? What bill collectors?" optimism about your finances?

Need a hint? What's the opposite of splurge? (Cough.) Budget, scrimp, save. (Cough.)

If you can't bear the thought of letting your charging arm get flabby from disuse, then you'll feel the least money worries when pulling out the cards for lesser-priced items or when caving to your progesterone-induced junk food cravings and hitting the 7-Eleven to buy a chili dog and blue Slurpee.

Career

As go-it-alone testosterone continues to decrease, you're in a team spirit kind of mood. And you make a valuable addition to any group. That's because, while it's true that your brain skills are on their way to the low end of their cycles, they're still only a mere three days past their Superwoman peak. What's more, you're still in your left brain, which makes you a whiz at analyzing reports, data, and fact checking. Plus, as you make the transition to your imaginative right brain, you're getting occasional brilliant flashes of creative insight.

As if all that weren't enough, you've got one more benefit to offer—the ability to handle pressure in the midst of any crisis. Your team can thank progesterone for that one. This hormone is blunting your stress response, which helps you keep your cool under any circumstance. Except, of course, when someone pushes your noradrenaline buttons. Which means you'll be able handle emergencies, such as the surprise visit from your company's biggest client, a system-wide computer failure, and the assistant who mistakenly shredded the only copy of the presentation you needed to make today, all without breaking a sweat. But if you come back from the ladies' room to find that your cubicle mate has eaten all your microwave popcorn, you might just have to staple his tongue to his Dilbert mouse pad.

Energy

VH1 Classics has more of a pull on you than MTV2. And the idea of joining the cast of Stomp isn't as appealing as, say, going for a leisurely stroll. But you still have the energy and endurance to be talked into yet another late night at the office by your passive-aggressive boss, pick up your clothes at the dry cleaner, come home and cook dinner, accidentally burn dinner, call up for takeout, and fall asleep in front of a late night talk show.

Hormone sensitive? Then you've still got the energy and endurance to make it through the same busy day. But your sensitivity to progesterone has you falling asleep by the time the ten o'clock news comes on instead.

Diet

Have you already given in to the progesterone-fueled temptation to nosh on sweets, salts, carbs, fats, and comfort foods? That means you'll be craving even more as the days go by. Which means it's probably time to make room on the shelves for all the Krispy Kremes and microwave popcorns you'll be needing.

On a diet and trying to resist the progesterone munchies? Not caving to junk food can help keep cravings to a minimum. But if you're hit with a particularly strong yearning for the bad stuff, taking a ten-minute walk can beat it into submission.

Because progesterone makes your blood sugar sensitive, you'll likely feel hungry every three to four hours. If you ignore your body's urgings to eat, you could become irritable, dizzy, or lightheaded, and get a headache. Snacking or eating five or six small meals throughout the day can prevent this, keeping your blood sugar more stable.

Add more fiber to your diet. Order a side salad. Eat a fiber-rich cereal. Or munch on a high-fiber cookie. It's not as tasty as a Pepperidge Farm, but it will help stave off progesterone-induced constipation.

Reality Check

Mood

You know how you forget all about some celebrities till their *E! True Hollywood Story* airs or they move into *The Surreal Life* house? Well, issues in your life are a lot like those forgotten stars—they seem to just pop up out of the blue.

Thing is, just like those oft-neglected B, C, and D listers, these problems were there all along. You simply didn't notice them. That's because, during the first half of your cycle, rising estrogen and testosterone were putting a positive spin on the people and events around you. But since Day 14, decreasing estrogen and testosterone have had you seeing life in a more realistic light. And by now you're starting to see situations as they really are rather than how you'd like them to be.

The result? Well, the result could be as mild as you realizing your roommate's 2:00 A.M. nude bongo playing is a lot less hip Bohemian artist, and a lot more of a reason

155

to kick him out. Or it could be as intense as realizing that you're really gay. Or you like karaoke.

Oh sure, some of the discoveries will be jarring. Coming out as a karaoke lover is hard on everyone at first. But if your cycle was all just optimism and glossing over issues, your life would never improve. It's the reality-check phase of your cycle that inspires you to take action to better your situation.

As estrogen and testosterone descend, you also continue to deal with pre-PMS hormone withdrawal symptoms—such as heart palpitations, a down-in-the-doldrums mood, weepiness, lack of confidence, and noradrenaline temper flares. But there's good news: Tomorrow estrogen and testosterone will rise again, putting an end to pre-PMS symptoms.

Till then, cocooning progesterone is bringing out the homebody in you. You may feel the urge to spend more time at home tidying up, trying new decorating ideas, or catching up on all those TiVo'd *Malcom in the Middle*s you missed during the first half of your cycle.

Sure-fire serotonin booster

Do some jumping jacks, take a swim, do yoga, or get your body moving any other way. Research shows that practically any form of exercise increases serotonin.

Mind

Your brain skills move from the high point to the midpoint of their cycle as cognition-enhancing estrogen and testosterone tumble. These brain skills remain at the midpoint till Day 22. So if there was something super-intelligent you were planning to do, say, mapping the genome of your pet cat, it'll still be easiest for the next seven days. After that, you might have to use your crib notes.

Thinking

While in the middle of your cognitive cycle, you can still concentrate, absorb new information, and make decisions. You just won't be able to do them while simultaneously juggling fire, painting your nails, and calling for an appointment for a Swedish massage, as you could during your high hormone days.

Memory

As your powers of recall fade from superhuman to just human, you'll still be able to remember names, dates, and faces. But your boy-toy might be able to get away with you forgetting about his promise to give the dog a bath.

Verbal

Progesterone continues to put a gap between your thoughts and the words coming out of your mouth. And your lexicon shrinks by a couple more words today. Slow-you-down progesterone also has you doing less speaking and more listening. So anyone who's been trying to interrupt your high estrogen/testosterone chatter with boring stories about her precocious kids or the intricate details of his last surgery may now thank your hormones for the ear time.

The side of your brain highlighted today?

Left brain to right brain: Transition—it happens all the time. A hairy caterpillar transforms into a beautiful butterfly. A tadpole transforms into frog. Madonna transforms into a married, middle-aged mother of two who creepily Frenches twenty-two-year-old girls to revive her waning career.

So, too, are you in transition, shifting from your analyzing and logical left brain to your creative and intuitive right brain.

Sure, there are benefits to being in either side. During your left brain phase you can swing a mean level and measure furniture to within a fraction of a millimeter. During your right brain phase it's a snap to dream up creative ways to get back at your neighbor for waking you up at 5:00 A.M. with the leaf blower. But when you're in the middle of a transition? You get the best of both worlds—logical wisdom mixed with flashes of ingenious insight.

Romance

If you're in a relationship . . .

Pity your boy. He's still scratching his head wondering why the dirty socks that have been piled in the corner the past two weeks suddenly bother you now. Poor thing, he simply doesn't understand that after the rose-colored glasses come off, that pile of smelly socks is less a charming personal quirk and a lot more grounds for separation.

Are there other problems in paradise? You—and no doubt he—will find out today as plunging estrogen and testosterone highlight the problems rather than the strengths in your relationship.

Did your guy pass the low estrogen and testosterone test and it turns out he has no faults whatsoever? Then progesterone has you rewarding him with nurturing kindness. You want to make him home-cooked meals, wipe that home-cooked sauce off his chin, and feed him with a flying airplane fork.

With wears-the-pants testosterone on the decline, you're also handing the remote over to your guy, letting him pick what to have for dinner, and generously letting him believe that he's making at least a few of the decisions in your relationship.

If you're single . . .

You're looking at your single's status and feeling doubtful. You don't have the high estrogen and testosterone confidence you'll find a mate that you had during the first half of the month. This is a temporary feeling, of course, as by Day 2 you know that the real reason George Clooney put off marriage was because he was waiting for you to say yes.

Sex

Your libido hits a serious lull and daydreams are more G- than X-rated as testosterone continues to take a dive and progesterone continues to plug up available testosterone receptors in your brain.

If you decide to take advantage of the few sparks of lust that come over you today, then you may want to get an extra set of batteries for the vibrator or tell your guy he should be prepared for more than just a quickie. While achievable, orgasms take minutes longer to reach than during the first half of your cycle. Your nipples and clitoris are less sensitive. And you're more easily distracted by sights, sounds, smells, and bad touches—for instance, his scratchy two-day beard growth that feels as if it's power sanding your cheek down to the bone. Ironically, while it takes longer to reach climax, plunging estrogen is slowing your lubrication just when you need it most. So patience and a bottle of personal lube may be needed.

And what about the quality of the orgasms themselves? Well, they're still worth going for. They're simply less "Oh! Oh! Oh!" and more "Oh!"

Money

Slipping out that credit card to buy a pricey luxury item? Forget it. Receding estrogen and testosterone totally nark you out. Before you know it, worry and guilt over finances come marching in like terrifying storm troopers of debt.

However, that probably still won't stop you from over-spending on things like new clothes, a haircut, or a top-of-the-line skin blemish cream. At least not while decreasing estrogen and testosterone are feeding your sense of self-doubt about your appearance. Because, let's face it—getting rid of a zit trumps guilt any day.

Career

Estrogen- and testosterone-induced spin control—it can make even the most life force–sucking job seem worth the three-zeros-short paycheck.

And now that decreasing estrogen and testosterone are stopping the spin cycle? Overtime no longer seems like an opportunity to demonstrate what a hard worker you are; it's the thing keeping the dark circles under your eyes and Juan Valdez in pesos. The company policy banning jeans, sneakers, and T-shirts no longer feels like a plan to promote an air of professionalism; instead, it's clearly a devious way to trick unsuspecting interviewees into believing they'll be paid a high enough wage to be able to afford dress clothes. And when Larry from the mailroom complains about the boss, rather than offer up a polite smile and an it-could-be-worse shrug, you're giving a conspiratorial nod and signing his petition to get a cappuccino machine in the employee lounge.

But no matter what kind of slap-in-the-face realizations you have about your job, your work product doesn't suffer. In fact, as you transition from the left brain to the right, you're becoming equally adept at analyzing reports and data and at coming up with ingenious solutions and out-of-the-box ideas.

While you don't mind going it alone, as long as the other people don't work your last noradrenaline-frayed nerve, you're happiest being part of a team. That's because decreasing testosterone has you less interested in leading and being the decision maker and more interested in the comfort of having someone else call the shots.

What's more, progesterone is making you sedate and less likely to initiate conversation, which has the team believing you're a patient listener who's sincerely interested in what they have to say. The fact that you're really mentally going over the list of munchies you'll be picking up on the way home to feed your progesterone cravings can be your little secret.

Energy

Okay, there's no denying it now. Your energy and endurance are taking a direct hit. But with estrogen and testosterone plunging and progesterone continuing to work its tranquilizing effect on you, it's hardly been a recipe for kick-ass enthusiasm and twenty-four-hour pep. Oh, you'll still be able to get through your usual routine. But you'll probably be yawning through that after-hours party.

If you're hormone sensitive, you're feeling about as energized as a Smiths song. Eating iron-rich foods and taking ten-minute naps can help maintain your stamina and help you make it through the end of your day. But you'll probably be asking for a rain check on that after-hours party.

Diet

Giving in to progesterone cravings is like giving in to the urge to have sex. Once you do it, you just want more. And you want to try it in different places. And with different people. And with different types of rubber outfits on.

On a diet, but fell off the sweets, salts, carbs, fats, and comfort food wagon? When the inevitable next craving hits, go for a ten-minute walk. It'll help reduce the yearning to a less all-consuming level.

Eat small meals every three to four hours to stabilize your blood sugar that's being made more sensitive by progesterone. And keep eating high fiber foods to prevent constipation that progesterone causes.

Transition Out of Pre-PMS

Mood

At some point today, the symptoms of pre-PMS disappear and—oh, let's face it, that's all the information you really wanted to know.

But in case you are still reading . . .

Till this transition happens, you continue to experience bouts of estrogen and testosterone withdrawal symptoms—such as anxiety, palpitations, the blues, a lack of self-confidence, and insecurity. And noradrenaline will still be trying to zing you with every traffic jam and computer crash.

Once estrogen and testosterone do rise, however, you can wave buh-bye to withdrawal symptoms. And how will you know they've started their upward swing? That you've gone a whole hour without a single mood swing will be a tipoff. That you don't feel like throwing your Pilates ball through the window when your roommate announces she doesn't have her share of the rent will be another.

Here's a bummer though: Estrogen and testosterone may be back on the upswing and doing wonders for stabilizing your mood, but they're not bringing all that supercharged optimism, confidence, and extroversion with them as they did the first half of your menstrual cycle. Oh, it's not their fault. It's party-pooping progesterone that's putting a cap on all the excitement. Its job is to keep your womb safe and sound just in case your egg got fertilized in the past few days. So it's doing all it can to persuade you to stay away from risky adventures, such as snowboarding and extreme office chair racing.

Progesterone would be so much happier if you were, say, at home baking cupcakes, knitting a scarf, or thumbing through the latest copy of *Us*. Or, if you must go out, it would prefer you stuck with close friends and family and avoid that whole date-swapping party altogether.

Mind

Your brain skills are like the careers of *Hollywood Squares* celebrity guests—they're not totally at the top, but they haven't hit rock bottom yet, either.

Thinking

Some might say you have the deep concentration of a professional eyebrow waxer. That's your progesterone— its calming properties make you appear as though you're paying attention for longer periods of time. But, of course, you could be thinking about the hunky guy in the apartment next door you've been meaning to ask on a date. If people think you're paying more attention, why let on?

Day 15 Day 16 Day 17 Day 18 Day 19 Day 20 Day 21

Memory

You might still be able to remember details and names you picked up in the last few days, but the current locations of your keys and glasses are a mystery.

Verbal

As progesterone increases, you're experiencing more verbal trip-ups. No biggie, since rising progesterone is also dampening your urge to chat, anyway.

The side of your brain highlighted today?

Left brain to right brain: As you get closer to Day 20, your right brain influence becomes stronger. As for left brain logic, with right brain creativity inspiring you to come up with inventive ways to do everything, from making an omelet to recording your voicemail greeting, you'll hardly miss it.

Romance

If you're in a relationship . . .

Did yesterday's reality check reveal any problems in your relationship? Then your reaction to them today is being influenced by your sensitivity to progesterone.

If you're not hormone sensitive and the problems aren't as big as, say, finding out he's a serial bank robber or—gosh forbid—a former male cheerleader, progesterone has you calm and serene, so you're not overly concerned about the problems. You know the issues are there, but you're like, "Hey, no relationship is perfect."

If you're hormone sensitive, progesterone has you feeling blue, so you're likely feeling bummed about even minor issues—for instance, that he's not making enough of an effort to help around the house, or it's been three days since he changed his underwear and that he's far too comfortable with that. These problems might seem to be overwhelming, insurmountable, or complete deal breakers.

Are you lucky enough to not have any problems in your relationship? Then progesterone has you showering nurturing kindness on your man. You're making him take his vitamins, insisting he eat the nutritious breakfast you whipped up for him, and putting a Batman Band-Aid on his boo-boo.

Not only that, but even though testosterone is back on the rise, you're still letting him call the shots in your relationship—what kind of snacks to buy, what movie to go see, and which video game he should play while you look on with feigned interest. That's not so much a reward for good behavior as it is progesterone blocking the testosterone that would normally increase your desire to be in control. But you can tell him it's a reward if it keeps him from forgetting to take out the trash or change his boxers.

If you're single . . .

When estrogen and testosterone begin to rise, the worry you may have experienced these past few pre-PMS days over not being able to find a guy wanes. Which gives you time to reconsider that billboard ad before your check clears.

Sex

Testosterone may be on the rise today, but progesterone is like a V-chip blocking your NC-17 libido. So you're not feeling the sexy effect you did from increasing testosterone during the first half of your cycle. As a result, your sex drive is low, your nipples and clitoris are less sensitive, it takes longer to orgasm, and the orgasms you do have pale in comparison to your high testosterone days.

You could try testosterone boosters—such as drinking caffeine, playing a game you're sure you'll win, or entering a competition. And you could try drinking a glass of wine if you're not sensitive to rising progesterone, since alcohol can also add to a blue mood. However, the effect on your sex drive will likely be mild because progesterone is plugging up the receptor cells needed to make testosterone work.

Oh, you may feel like spending your day cursing sex-squashing progesterone. But you could use that same time and energy to summon up what little sex drive you have and use progesterone's Zen calmness to explore tantric sex or tantric masturbation. It'll certainly make for interesting dinner conversation when you and the gals get together to catch up.

Money

If your finances were a game of tic-tac-toe, they'd be a draw. That's because spend-loving estrogen and testosterone may be on the rise but their effect is being cut off by play-it-safe progesterone, so you don't feel like splurging. But if you do pull out the cards today, at least you won't have all the messy guilt and worry that comes with decreasing estrogen and testosterone. Which pretty much greenlights that hot pink Versace jacket you've been eyeing.

Career

You're still seeing work in a more realistic light. Which means Al from sales still has the world's worst coffee breath. And your boss is still an arrogant know-it-all whose Match.com profile that's been surreptitiously going around the office still seems as made up as a Jayson Blair article.

But how you react to issues at work is influenced by your sensitivity to progesterone:

If you're not sensitive, then progesterone has you feeling serene, which is happily blunting the frustration over the problems at work. You acknowledge them, but you're like, "Hey, doesn't every job have its faults?"

If you're hormone sensitive, progesterone has you feeling down in the dumps, which has you bummed over problems at work. You can't even understand why you thought you'd want a raise or promotion just a week ago. Not when it feels as if you're ready to post your resume on Monster.com and jump at the first offer that comes along.

Whatever your progesterone-induced reaction to your job, you're still a major player at work. That's because, as you continue to make the transition from your left to right brain, you're adept at both logical tasks and brainstorming creative ideas.

Testosterone may be on the rise, but it doesn't reach the leadership levels it did during the first half of your cycle, so you prefer working in teams with someone else making the decisions. And with estrogen rising, even your most annoying coworker won't unwittingly step on any noradrenaline landmines.

Energy

Energizing estrogen and testosterone rise today. However, so does sedating progesterone. The result? You'll have the endurance to get through a hectic, to-do filled day. You'll just be doing it at a speed that makes a turtle look Hemi-powered.

Hormone sensitive? Then progesterone has you sedate, sleepy, and thinking that there could be worse things than getting strung out on Red Bull.

Diet

"Sweets, salts, carbs, fats, and comfort foods are yummy. You want them. You really, really want them," progesterone coos. If you give in to the temptation, you'll want them even more. If you don't give in, progesterone will have less power over you and your grocery-shopping list.

If you already gave in but want to stop the junk food madness, going for a ten-minute walk when cravings hit will decrease the urge. And putting ten blocks between you and that can of Pringles can't hurt either.

To combat progesterone-related blood sugar sensitivity, continue eating five or six small meals a day or snacking every three to four hours to keep dizziness and the crankies away.

And to combat progesterone-related constipation, continue including fiber in your diet—for instance, maybe have a tasty sandwich on whole wheat bread. Or, if high fiber foods aren't your thing, simply pop a high fiber supplement.

More salt, less bloat

How sinister! Just when progesterone has you craving salty snacks—hot, buttered popcorn, pretzels, and French fries—it's also making you bloat like a puffer fish the second a single grain of the white stuff passes over your lips. What can you do? Switch to sea salt! Because it has a different chemical makeup, it doesn't cause bloat like table salt does![1]

A Time to Address Important Issues

Mood

Estrogen and testosterone are on the rise today. While this usually means good news, don't IM your buddy list and tell everyone to meet up at your house with the margarita mix just yet. Before estrogen and testosterone can reach the party levels of Days 1 through 13, progesterone storms in like a home-too-soon parent, putting the kibosh on any fun activities (read: illegal, dangerous, and has the potential to show up on *www.theSmokingGun.com* right before your bid for presidency), and sends you to bed early.

Why does progesterone have to be such a total square? It can't help it. Its role is to be the ultimate parent watching over your uterus. It's thickening your uterine lining to give your egg a better hold in case fertilization occurred. And it's doing its best to keep you from going out partying and risking a disco-related injury. It'd be much happier if you just sat safely on your egg in your nest eating for two.[1] Or at least hung out on the couch watching the Oxygen channel and scarfing down Devil Dogs with abandon. And in case you get any other ideas, progesterone is persuading you to stay put by making you as sedated as Rush Limbaugh and too hungry to go further than ten feet from the fridge.

If you're hormone sensitive, progesterone may make you feel blue, unsure of yourself, and weepy. Certainly not the makings of a good time. But if it keeps you from going to that after-hours club, progesterone feels that its work is done.

And what about rising estrogen? Is it bringing nothing to the table? Oh, it's bringing it. In fact, it's bringing you one of the best gifts of all: happiness-in-a-hormone serotonin. That means you'll be seeing a lot less of rage-against-the-machine noradrenaline and feeling lots more good vibrations.

So tell the boy toy it's safe to come out of hiding and join you on the couch. And to bring a plate of fresh-baked cinnamon buns with him.

Mind

Estrogen and testosterone rise, but they don't do much to bounce brain skills up a notch. That's progesterone's fault. It muffles the usual brain-sharpening effect of these two hormones. But don't threaten to kick progesterone's ass just yet. This hormone is also the one that's keeping you calm and sedate. And that translates into scoring extra points for looking like you've got better listening skills— even if you really are just daydreaming about your next trip to Dunkin' Donuts. So it's all good.

Thinking

Exams, reports, coming up with a new way to shuffle cards before the girls' poker game tonight—all easy as your focus, learning, and decision-making skills hover around the midpoint of their phases. Now, winning at the *Who Wants to Be a Millionaire?* board game night—that's gonna need a bit of extra effort. But being able to do your victory in-your-face dance will make it sooo worth it.

Memory

There could be worse things than having your memory at the middle of its cycle. When Day 28 comes around, you'll know what those are.

Verbal

Quieting progesterone has you less interested in chatting. Maybe it's this hormone's way of hiding the fact that, the higher it goes, the more stumbley your speech becomes.

The side of your brain highlighted today?

Left brain to right brain: True confession time. Do you still dream of one day going back to school? Do you wonder if you'll ever start your own business? Do you see more red flags popping up about your mate than are on the Grand Slalom course?

As progesterone continues to push you into an introspective right brain phase, deep-down concerns and issues that you've put off dealing with begin to bubble to the surface once again. It's not that these issues weren't important during the high-estrogen days of your cycle. You were simply too busy chasing boys and launching your career to take time to think about them. Now sluggish progesterone has you busier thinking than doing.

These concerns and issues will remain prominent throughout the rest of your cycle. But today through Day 22 is the perfect opportunity to confront them. That's because rising estrogen and testosterone are keeping your mood stable. By the time Day 23 comes around and PMS hits, these problems feel bigger and more out of control.[2]

Romance

If you're in a relationship . . .

Is your mate longing for the days when he could drink straight out of the milk carton, leave orange Cheez Doodle dust all over your keyboard, and change the channel right in the middle of *The View*—and you'd still think he was the greatest guy, like, ever? He can put the blame squarely on your progesterone. It's stopping rising estrogen and testosterone from hiding all his faults behind an impermeable wall of optimism as they so conveniently did on Days 1 through 13.

Your introspective right brain loves a good mulling over, so no doubt you're pondering your boy toy's recently highlighted shortcomings. However, it's your sensitivity to progesterone that will determine the plan of action you decide to take.

If you're not hormone sensitive, mellowing progesterone has you thinking his problems may qualify him as a fixer-upper, but you've got your tool belt and you're ready for the job. If you're hormone sensitive, depressing progesterone is making even his smallest problems feel too massive an undertaking to even attempt fixing. And it may just seem easier to switch to a new guy altogether.

Is your guy utterly faultless? Remembers every special occasion without prompting? Gives you thoughtful birthday gifts that he bought weeks in advance? Even dusts your altar to Brad Pitt? Then progesterone has you smothering him with motherly nurturing. Perhaps you'll scrub his back for him in the shower, make him a hot bowl of chicken soup, or offer to hold the tissue while he blows his nose.

You also continue to let your guy make many of the decisions in the relationship. That's because progesterone continues to block the testosterone that would normally increase your desire to be in control. But if letting him choose a new ring tone for the phone and decide which kind of toilet paper you should buy makes him feel like The Man, why quibble?

If you're single . . .

If your cat isn't enough of a nurturing outlet for you, progesterone likely has you craving a relationship and all its co-dependent trappings right about now.

Sex

Thoughts of sex are about as frequent as a zero balance on your credit cards. Your nipples and clitoris are less sensitive to touch. It takes minutes longer to reach orgasm than on a high testosterone day. And the orgasms you do reach are mere shadows of the knee-knockers you had in the first half of your cycle. Is there any reason to break out the condoms at all?

Truth? Yes. For starters, it's all relative. An orgasm during the first half of your menstrual cycle is like Disneyland. It's big, it's bold, at points you're flying through the air. But you don't stop going to your small neighborhood amusement park just because you had a wild time with the Mouse, right? So, sure, the orgasm isn't as intense. And, sure, it doesn't radiate all over your body like it did just a week ago. But it still feels pretty good.

Plus, having regular orgasms—whether self-induced or partner-induced—is actually healthy. No lie! Orgasms produce oxytocin, which helps get you to sleep, dopamine, which alleviates stress, and even estrogen.[3] Yes, estrogen. And the more of that you produce, the happier you feel.

Money

With forget-about-bills estrogen and testosterone on the rise, guilt and worry over spending is low. However, you still probably won't feel like heading to Macy's for a buying bender. That's progesterone's fault. It's blunting the usual shop-till-you-drop urges that accompany rising estrogen and testosterone in the first half of your cycle.

But this doesn't mean your credit cards are going to get a chance to cool off. Fact is, as progesterone ushers you into a nurturing phase, it's making it harder to resist splurging on housewares, home accents, furniture, and anything else that will make your home feel cozier.

Career

Creativity, writing skills, and team spirit. You've got the makings for joining the *SNL* writing staff or for coming up with a new product, department, or project at work. Totally your call.

As the reality of your life continues to come into tighter focus, you see your place of employment as it really is, rather than what you remember from the help-wanted ad when you first applied. If you're not sensitive to progesterone, then you're okay with what you see. Oh sure, the vending machine is out of Milk Duds. The coffee is the cheap stuff. And you're pretty sure you're cubicle is slowly decreasing in size each day. But you can deal.

If you're sensitive to rising progesterone, you'd better remember to erase the history on your Internet browser before the boss discovers that you're hunting around for jobs with the competition.

Energy

If you're not sensitive to hormones, rising progesterone has your energy winding down like the number of remaining Ace of Base fans. Estrogen and testosterone may continue to be on the rise, but the only real help they're giving is that they're stopping progesterone from making you so sedate that you fall asleep in your Fruity Pebbles.

If you're sensitive to hormones, rising estrogen and testosterone give you even less of a help. The more progesterone you produce, the tireder you get. Tireder? Yeah, tireder. Do you really have enough energy to look it up?

Diet

Including lots of fiber in your diet? Yes. Eating every three to four hours? Yes. Giving in to progesterone-driven cravings for sweets, salts, carbs, fats, and comfort foods? Only if you're really sure you want to. Because once you start, just as with cocaine, cigarettes, and shopping on eBay, it's so much harder to stop.

Taking a ten-minute walk to reduce cravings after you've given in to temptation? Definitely.

Switch to the Right Brain

Mood

Something important happens today. Michael Jackson finally admits to having plastic surgery—like, a thousand times? Size 0 models figure out they can save a fortune on boob jobs, butt implants, and collagen lip injections just by eating a sandwich? Britney Spears realizes that if she only stopped dancing so much she could catch her breath and stop lip-synching?

Even more important: You complete the transition from your logical left brain to your creative right brain.

Okay, it's not like you didn't see this coming. You've been transitioning to your right brain phase since you entered the second phase of your cycle on Day 14. But today progesterone finally pushes you over the line and has your logical and analytical left brain taking a back seat to your emotional and creative right brain. This means for the next 14 days reason will be overshadowed by senti-ment, practicality will make way for what feels right, and facts will be replaced by hunches, gut instinct, and what-ever your online psychic tells you.

Progesterone is still dominating your days, so you're feeling a bit slowed down and sedate. If you're hormone sensitive, then progesterone also has you teary, blue, or possibly even depressed. And that's even before turning on the Lifetime channel.

And what about estrogen and testosterone? Progesterone may be hogging the spotlight, but estrogen and testosterone are still behind the scenes doing their best to keep your mood stable by producing uplifting serotonin and dopamine.

Mind

Estrogen and testosterone continue to rise, but progesterone squashes their effect, leaving your brain skills at the midpoint. Not a bad place to be. Especially when you consider you've got your creative right brain to rely on now to pick up the slack.

Thinking

Practically anything is achievable as concentration, comprehension, and decision making are at the midpoint of their cycles. Some things might require a little more effort—such as coming up with a new Middle East peace plan or getting a new CD out of its packaging in under thirty minutes. Some things will require a little less effort—such as doing long division or reading *The Globe*.

Memory

Your recall is no Day 13. But your brain is a veritable fact sponge compared to Day 28. Which means, you may not be able to recall the kabillionth decimal of pi. But you will be able to remember where you put important files and that tonight's a premier of yet another *CSI* spinoff.

Verbal

If it feels as if someone is pressing a few too many space bars between your words, that's progesterone's fault. As it rises, it continues to add a few hesitations in your speech.

The side of your brain highlighted today?

Right brain: During this right brain introspective phase, important life issues continue to dominate your thoughts. You may be wondering about your relationship, career, family, goals, or what to change the ring tone to on your cell.

Got a decision to make today? You're using your right brain emotions and intuition to guide you.[1] For instance, need to pick a restaurant? You base your choice on whether the ambiance makes you feel at home and the wait staff makes you feel welcome, rather than on location, price, or quality of food. Need to pick out a new cell phone? You make your choice based on the color of the light-up buttons. Have to decide on a new Internet provider? You see who the I Ching recommends. Remember when making decisions used to be boring?

Romance

If you're in a relationship . . .

Does your relationship have issues? If you're not sensitive to hormones, then mellowing progesterone has you acknowledging your guy's flaws and taking pity on him. You know he can't be perfect. At least not till you're finished whipping him into shape.

If you're sensitive to hormones, then downhearted-inducing progesterone has you feeling a bit of self-pity. You can't understand why he's not perfect. Especially after all the time you've spent trying to whip him into shape.

Are you in the perfectest relationship, like, ever? Give yourselves a little back patting, remember not to flaunt it too much in front of your friends with less-perfect relationships, and then feel free to give in to progesterone's urgings to nurture your man.

If you're single . . .

Progesterone is kicking up your need to nurture. And that has you craving a relationship and everything that comes with it—intimacy, companionship, and someone else to blame.

Sex

Progesterone goes up. Libido, sensitivity of your nipples and clitoris, ease of climax, and intensity of orgasm go down. It's not a pretty scenario.

But if you do want to make the most of the few sparks of arousal that pass over you today by going for the O, then you'll be rewarded with calming oxytocin, stress-relieving dopamine, and mood-enhancing estrogen.

Money

With nesting progesterone continuing to push you to make your home more beautiful, you may feel the need for an emergency run to Pottery Barn for a decorative throw rug. Or if you're in a pinch for a decorative fix but can't leave the house, you might feel like hitting Overstock.com for some wall sconces and a nifty takeout menu holder. Go ahead and splurge. Rising estrogen and testosterone promise they'll keep the guilties away, no matter how many toaster cozies you buy.

Career

Your boss ranting about how to boost sales, cut expenses, or keep employees from downloading virus-infected games onto the company computer system? (True, she rants about so much, who can keep track?) But if she's boiling about a problem that needs, say, a little creativity and out-of-the-box thinking, this is your chance to impress. Imagination? You've got it. Problem solving? Child's play. A raise? Possibly in the works if you can get your inventive ideas across to Ms. Decibel in between bouts of shouting.

Perhaps you're better off proposing your suggestions in a memo. That way you don't have to wait for her to take a breath to speak up. And, besides, during your right brain phase, you're much more eloquent in written prose than spoken word, anyway.

Still seeing the workplace as, well, a workplace and not the challenging, fun, potentially mate-finding place where you spend ~~50 percent~~ ~~60 percent~~ 75 percent of your life? Yes. But if you're not sensitive to progesterone, then you're okay with it. You know you have to take the good with the bad. And you're pretty sure the guy from Accounts Payable is recently single.

If you're sensitive to progesterone, then you may be tempted to save all those creative suggestions for your new employer. Who, with so many feelers out, you hope to be hearing from any day now.

Energy

The dishes. Vacuuming. Line dancing. (Things you won't feel like doing even if you're not sensitive to sedating progesterone.)

Waking up. Staying awake. Staying awake longer. (Things you won't feel like doing if you are sensitive to sedating progesterone.)

Ah, sedating progesterone. Responsible for keeping the twelve-Starbucks-per-square-mile ratio intact.

Diet

The road to hell is paved with good intentions. The high-way to hell, however, is paved with corn chips, soda, and chocolate chip cookies, and it has McFood rest stops at every mile. Guess which one you're on?

Progesterone continues to have you craving sweets, salts, carbs, fats, and comfort foods. More so if you've already succumbed to temptation. Less so if you don't indulge at all and take ten-minute walks at every craving.

Include lots of fiber to prevent progesterone-induced constipation. And eat every three to four hours to prevent light-headedness and the irritability that come with your increased sensitivity to blood sugar during your proges-terone phase.

Mellowed Out

Mood

You don't so much walk as slowly saunter. Your words come at an unhurried pace. Even your laugh sounds leisurely. Are you a gal whose got lots of progesterone coursing through her brain? Or a gal who's cool in a low-key, Macy Gray kinda way? Okay, it's progesterone. But why let on?

If you're not sensitive to hormones, progesterone is making you feel tranquil and laid back. Even for the most thrilling of events, it's hard to muster much excitement. Friends might mistake your subdued reaction about landing your first movie role, making partner in the firm, or having your boyfriend propose as events not worth celebrating. Not true. Your enthusiastic reaction is simply confined to doing your happy dance on the inside.

If you're sensitive to hormones, progesterone is keeping you quiet, reserved, and unapologetically serene in the face of all things exciting. But it also has you lethargic, down in the dumps, and weepy. Turning on the WE channel or watching practically anything starring Shirley MacLaine can turn this mild sobfest into the full-blown bawling of ditched-prom-date proportions.

If you're taking monophasic hormone contraceptives that dole out a constant amount of progesterone, you'll feel a bit slower. However, this effect will likely be milder because your progesterone doesn't reach the high peak that natural hormones and biphasic and triphasic hormone contraceptives do.

But no matter what your hormone sensitivity or which hormone contraceptives you take, rising estrogen continues to try to break on through progesterone's Valium-like effects and imbue you with the feel-good brain chemicals serotonin and dopamine. And rising testosterone tries to make you feel safer and more secure about your body—a toughie on any day, but even more so on a day when progesterone-induced snack cravings are near their peak and bloating and premenstrual acne have made it clear that they're moving in, setting up their beach chairs, and sticking around till Day 28.

What rising estrogen and testosterone won't manage to do, however, is amp you up to the risk-taking, extroversion levels that they did in the first half of your cycle. That's progesterone's fault. Under the assumption that you might have a fertilized egg to protect, it's trying to keep you far away from daring adventures and unfamiliar places that don't have the fire exit signs clearly marked. As a result, you feel safest and most comfortable hanging out with close friends or family in spots that you consider your "usual" haunts—such as the mall, your favorite café, or the front table at Chippendale's.

Mind

Even as cognitive-enhancing estrogen and testosterone rise, progesterone keeps your brain skills at the midpoint of their cycle. Yeah, it's a gyp. But what're you gonna do?

Thinking

While your hormones are in the middle of their cycle, focus, ability to absorb information, and decision making are also in the middle. You're not at the top of your game. But you're not bottoming out either. And that alone deserves a bit of thanks.

Memory

While in the middle of your memory cycle, you're still able to recall most details with ease. Though facts about your bank balance and credit card limit may still elude you. But, really, don't those fall under the less-you-know-the-better category, anyway?

Verbal

Progesterone continues to inject pauses and stops into your sentences as it delays word recall and verbal response. It's not as noticeable though, since you're feeling like doing less talking, anyhow.

The side of your brain highlighted today?

Right brain: Ah, right brain phase—come for the ingenious solutions to any problem; stay for the creative way it can transform last season's Jelly bag into a stylish goldfish bowl.

You may feel like sitting and contemplating issues, problems, and the transcendental subtexts of Saturday morning cartoons while watching your fish swim happily about in the bag that used to house your lipstick samples and spare tongue stud. That's because pondering progesterone combines with your introspective right brain to make getting lost in thought practically your fallback position. The right brain isn't all about weighty issues, though. You'll also notice that your writing skills improve and you're more in touch with your feelings.

While right brainers tend to prefer piles and are comfortable surrounded by a flurry of Post-Its, nesting progesterone is pushing you to tidy up the house. The result? While your work area may be a blizzard of papers and notes, you might feel compelled to spend an hour getting the toilet to shine as brilliantly as the gold teeth on a gangsta.

Romance

If you're in a relationship . . .

Your honey has a few faults? If you're not sensitive to hormones, then your blasé mood from progesterone has you shrugging them off. You know he's got some negatives, but his positive qualities make up for them.

If you're sensitive to hormones, then your blue mood from progesterone has you overwhelmed with his faults.

And right about now you can't even remember what positive qualities led you to ever be attracted to him.

In a relationship with a Mr. Wonderful? Then nurturing progesterone has you wanting to baby him. However, he may draw the line at you mashing up his hot dogs and feeding him another meal with the flying airplane fork.

If you're single . . .

The progesterone-induced urge to nurture may have you longing for a mate to do all the kinds of care-taking things you do in a relationship—like cutting up his meat for him, scratching his back when it itches, and giving him lots of treats. But for now, your cat will be the happy beneficiary of all your nurturing impulses. Which may explain Fluffy's tendency to claw the hell out of any date you bring home.

Sex

Progesterone is keeping your sex drive low, decreasing the sensitivity in your nipples and clitoris, and making it take a long, long, long, long time to reach orgasm. The base of the mountain is littered with men who have helped you try. But once you reach it, you'll be glad you stuck it out. Your guy, however, may need an oxygen tank and a week off till you try again.

Money

You can never have too many decorative home accents. At least that's what nesting progesterone and Bed Bath & Beyond want you to believe.

Career

Strengths: Creativity, problem solving, brainstorming, writing.

Weaknesses: As if! You're an asset to any team that needs to come up with a brilliant idea or solution. And with your right brain surging, you're the go-to gal to put that great idea down on paper.

Do your boss and coworkers not recognize the creative genius that's standing right in front of them? If you're not sensitive to progesterone, then your cool mood has you taking it with a grain of salt. You figure it's their loss. And besides, whatever ideas they don't run with, you'll use to make your first million the second you're out of this job.

If you're sensitive to progesterone, your down mood may have you feeling slighted when colleagues don't use your amazing ideas. You figure if they can't see the awesomeness of your proposals, then they're obviously not very good at their jobs. In which case, it's only a matter of time before the company goes under, anyway, so you may as well get out while you still have your 401(k) intact.

Energy

Not sensitive to hormones? Then progesterone has you feeling calm, mellow, and Zen-like. But without having to figure out all those really hard koans.

Sensitive to hormones? Then progesterone has you tired, listless, and longing for a nap. Pretty much the same effect you get after spending thirty minutes trying to decipher what the hell Ozzy's saying.

Diet

Been indulging in sweets, salts, carbs, fats, and comfort foods? Then passing a bakery or fast food joint is an exercise in willpower. Looking down to see you polished off the whole box of cookies is scarily commonplace.

Been avoiding sweets, salts, carbs, fats, and comfort foods so far? Then you barely notice any cravings. Don't brag too much about it. Your dieting friends might feel compelled to sneak heavy cream into your skinny latté.

Did you start indulging but now want to stop? You know the drill—ten minutes of walking for every craving.

Continue to eat every three to four hours to level out your blood sugar, which will keep your mood up. And fiber is still a must during this progesterone phase. Unless your menstrual cycle just isn't the same without the monthly constipation and the heaviness, hemorrhoids, and yeast infections that come with it.

Day 22

The Calm Before the Storm

Mood

Today you amaze everyone with your ability to stay unruffled in the face of any crisis. A car crashes through the store you're shopping in? You barely muster a glance. Your roommate starts a kitchen fire while trying to flambé tofu? As you nonchalantly douse it with the fire extinguisher, you still find time to check your hair in the feng shui mirror above the stove. The "big boss" comes in for a surprise inspection? Everyone freaks. You? Puhleeze. Your unshakable serenity makes a yogi master look like an espresso whore.

You can tell everyone you're simply too together to let anything get to you. The truth, however, is that progesterone has you feeling wonderfully relaxed, calm, and centered. It's like you did an hour of meditation. But without having to sit still for an hour pretending not to be bored out of your freaking mind.

Progesterone's effects are most intense if your hormones are natural or if you take biphasic or triphasic contraceptives. A tad less so if you're taking monophasic hormone contraceptives, since your progesterone doesn't peak as high. A tad more so if you're sensitive to hormones, in which case, progesterone will have you feeling sluggish, depressed, and a bit weepy.

As for estrogen and testosterone, they peak for a second time in your cycle today. It could be a little less so if you're taking monophasic hormone contraceptives. But either way, these two hormones still don't reach the superconfident and extroverted levels of the first half of your cycle. To be fair though, estrogen and testosterone do have the premenstrual evil duo—bloating and acne—feverishly plotting against them now.

But it's really motherly progesterone that prevents peaking estrogen and testosterone from reaching the self-assured, adventurous levels of the first half of your cycle. That's because progesterone wants to keep you and what it believes could be your fertilized egg safe and sound and away from risky, bedlam-filled adventures, such as fashion magazine parties and extreme scrapbooking. Which is why cozier, more familiar settings make you happiest today. And even happier if they're within ordering distance to lots of comfort food just in case there's the remotest chance that you'll want to give in to a few of those many progesterone cravings.

Mind

Tomorrow estrogen and testosterone plunge, and take your brain skills down with them. That makes this the last day that your brain skills are at the midpoint of their cycle.

Thinking

Last exit till the low end of your concentration, learning skills, and decision-making abilities. 'Nuff said?

Memory

Sure, you may be able to remember dates, names, and facts today. But you might want to break out a notebook for the memory-sapping days ahead.

Verbal

Your speech is slower and there are a few pauses between your thoughts and the words coming out of your mouth. You can tell people it's for dramatic emphasis. But it's really progesterone causing a delay in word recall and verbal ability.

The side of your brain highlighted today?

Right brain: Creative solutions are as plentiful as grains of sand in a bathing suit bottom. Your guy always loses the remote? You crazy glue his beer bottle opener to it. Your roommate keeps sneaking your expensive hair products? You fill decoys with her cheap stuff. Your cat won't stop clawing the chair legs? You protect them by wrapping them with scratch 'n' sniff stickers. Oooo, furniture saving *and* room deodorizing.

Got something to contemplate or ponder, for example, the relevance of string theory or why you can't get adult-sized Underoos? Slow-you-down progesterone combines with your introspective right brain to set the stage for a good think.

Writing is easier to do during your right brain phase. So if you've been meaning to tell your state senator that you demand affordable healthcare or to send your letter calling for the return of Pepsi Blue, now would be a perfect time to do it.

Romance

If you're in a relationship . . .

Your sweetie flawed? If you're not sensitive to hormones, then you're like, "Whatevah. Even if he does insist on putting ketchup on practically everything I cook for him, it's all good."

Are you sensitive to hormones? Then you're totally focused on the latest made-for-TV movie where Mary-Ann just discovered that her daughter, whom she gave up for adoption, now lives across the street, but she can't say anything because the adoptive parents won't let her. So what else could possibly matter?

Is your sweetie as unflawed as a pint of Cherry Garcia? Then progesterone has your urge to nurture at a cycle-long high. You'll be trimming crusts off his PB & J sandwiches and wiping schmutz off his cheek with your thumb and some spittle before he has a chance to say "Ewww."

If you're single . . .

Progesterone likely has you craving a mate to coddle. Unless, of course, you're perfectly happy doting on Mr. Whiskers.

Sex

Hard work—it can get you lots of stuff: financial independence, a Ph.D., your own line of handmade lip balms in cosmetic stores around the country.

Same goes with sex. You can reach orgasm today. But with progesterone clogging up your testosterone receptors, it just takes a little hard work. Okay, a lotta hard work. Okay, your hand will cramp up and your boy toy's penis will likely fall off before it happens. But when you do reach it, it will be *sooo* worth it.

Money

Progesterone's keeping a lid on excited emotions. Which means enthusiastic salesmen and peppy infomercial hosts have little effect on you. Yet, oddly enough, just looking at potpourri dishes, designer pillow shams, and artsy wall hooks will have your charge cards virtually jumping out of your purse all by themselves.

That's your progesterone-induced nesting instinct kicking in. It's giving you the urge to buy whatever makes your home more beautiful, comfortable, and perfectly coordinated, right down to the last decorative glass bead.

And what do estrogen and testosterone have to say about all the splurging going on in the home furnishings department? They're still rising, which means guilt over spending is low. So if you really want to drop $79 for a set of coasters, they're not going to be the ones to stop you.

Career

Your boss sends you an urgent e-mail (despite the fact that she's a mere three feet from your cube and could holler faster than it takes to type, but, whatevah) and needs a brillianter than brilliant coverline/logo/ad campaign/product/excuse for why she hasn't gotten back to the client yet, and you're her go-to gal. Can you deliver? You bet! That's because you're deep into your right brain, where creativity is queen. You've got more ideas than a dead rock star has drugs listed in his autopsy report. And you're brainstorming with more ease than TV producers thinking up the next reality show plot twist.

During your right brain phase, it's easier to express yourself in writing than in spoken word. So if you plan to propose any of your imaginative ideas to the boss, you'll be more effective using interoffice e-mail than presenting them in person.

Did you put your suggestions in writing and your boss still shot them down? If you're not sensitive to progesterone, then you're in too much of a calm mood to let it get to you. Your attitude is if she didn't like these ideas, you've got plenty of others to clog up her inbox.

If you're sensitive to progesterone, your blue mood will likely have you feeling bummed at any sign of a no and make you hesitant to send other submissions your boss's way.

199

That's all right. By Day 2, you'll be feeling more optimistic and will still be in your creative right brain. (Which means you'll get your shot at clogging up your boss's inbox, too.)

Energy

Not sensitive to hormones? Then progesterone has you feeling about as subdued as a crowd at a Yanni concert. Sensitive to hormones? Then progesterone has you craving a nap pretty much the moment you wake up.

Diet

Ooey, gooey hot Pillsbury cinnamon rolls. Sinfully carb-rich, deep-fried McDonalds hash browns. Waffles smothered in butter and syrup with a side of crisp, salty bacon. If you've been indulging your cravings, then this list of comfort foods will have your mouth watering so much you probably won't be able to get to the end of this sentence before bolting off to the nearest vending machine for a craving fix.

Still reading? Then you've probably been staying far away from sweets, salts, carbs, fats, and comfort foods. Or you've been doing a lot of walking to chase away cravings.

Regardless of whether you indulge or resist temptation, you should still be eating lots of constipation-preventing fiber and chowing down about every three to four hours to keep your blood sugar level and the grouchies at bay.

Descent into PMS

PMS Alert

The biggest difference between PMS and pre-PMS is that the symptoms of hormone withdrawal during PMS are way more intense.[1] This is true regardless of whether your hormones are natural or you're taking hormone contraceptives.

However, the characteristics of your personal PMS depend a lot on whether your hormones are natural or which hormone contraceptives you take. Here's how it breaks down:

Are your hormones natural? If your egg wasn't fertilized during ovulation, from today to Day 28 you experience withdrawal from all three hormones—estrogen, testosterone, and progesterone.

Take hormone contraceptives with progesterone only? From today through Day 26 you experience withdrawal from just two hormones—estrogen and testosterone. When your progesterone runs out around Day 26, you'll be withdrawing from all three hormones till Day 28.

Take hormones with both estrogen and progesterone? Then you won't feel the full effects of PMS till around Day 26 when you reach the end of your hormones for this cycle. This doesn't mean you're completely off the hook till then, however. Many women who take hormone contraceptives with estrogen and progesterone report that they still experience PMS symptoms around this time of their cycle. Some researchers believe it may be because your body's other hormones and brain chemicals have cyclical fluctuations that mimic PMS symptoms. Other researchers speculate that a woman's own hormones may be breaking through and causing cycle fluctuations. Whatever the cause, you'll likely experience a milder version of PMS till your hormones run out on Day 26. Then you feel the full effects of estrogen, testosterone, and progesterone withdrawal till Day 28.

Are you making PMS worse?

You are if you drink caffeinated beverages from today through Day 23. That's because, no matter what your hormone sensitivity is, coffee, tea, Red Bull, Kahlua, and all other sources of caffeine can take whatever PMS symptoms you'd normally experience and supersize them. Mild anxiety turns into bone-vibrating jitters. Gentle sobbing turns into all-out wailing. Shades of sadness turn into gut-wrenching depression. And knowing what you do about noradrenaline, do you really want to give it a competitive edge? So skip the java and head for the juice joint instead.[2]

What's on TV?

From today to Day 28, you prefer sitcoms, funny movies, or any other kind of show that makes you laugh and helps you forget all about your premenstrual aches and pains.

Want a refresher on which withdrawing hormones are causing which symptom? Of course you do—how else will you know which hormone to put a voodoo curse on when you feel a withdrawal symptom approaching? Decreasing estrogen is the one that causes bouts of nervousness, anxiety, teariness, and the blues. Estrogen withdrawal also decreases mood-stabilizing serotonin, which spells the return of burst-on-the-scene noradrenaline. So if something irritates you—for instance, your guy spills coffee on your brand-new sofa—all you can really do is sit back and say, "Temper flare, meet boyfriend. Boyfriend, meet temper flare."

Testosterone withdrawal ushers in feelings of self-doubt about your appearance and abilities. No matter how many times you blow dry your hair or go over your report, it seems like a monkey could've done a better job. Or at least a male model.

Meanwhile, withdrawing progesterone has you weeping at just about anything.[3] A friend's engagement announcement. Commercials. A piece of lint. Stock up on tissues now and you won't have to resort to using the sleeves of your dry-clean-onlys to mop up running mascara.

Depending on your hormone sensitivity and which hormone contraceptive you take, these symptoms will be only mild and infrequent or they'll annoy you with more frequency and intensity than pop up ads on a porn site.

Some good news: No matter what your PMS is like, withdrawal symptoms aren't a constant. They're more like annoying tollbooths on the thruway of your cycle. You just try to pay your fare and get through as quickly as possible without dropping your quarters underneath the car.

Mood

In between withdrawal symptoms, your day is pretty low-key. Progesterone has you feeling mellow. And low levels of estrogen and testosterone have you feeling thoughtful and introspective. You're kinda like a folk singer, but without the acoustic guitar and marijuana conviction.

Because you never know when a withdrawal symptom is going to hit, you'll probably prefer sticking close to home, where things are familiar and somewhat predictable (but woe to the next-door neighbor who decides to throw a tub-thumping house party without your prior knowledge).

Feeling weepy?

Let the tears flow! Crying releases mood-lifting endorphins. That means before that final tear has melted the last of your mascara you'll already be feeling better![4]

The activities you'll enjoy the most are those that give a boost to decreasing serotonin and, subsequently, keep feisty noradrenaline in check. Such as? Anything that's guaranteed to be a good time and not annoying at all—curling up to a pint of Ben & Jerry's and a fashion mag, taking a soothing bubble while listening to your favorite CD, or indulging in a hot stone massage. Sigh. If only serotonin-boosting wasn't such hard work . . .

Sure-fire serotonin booster

Eat turkey, drink milk, or treat yourself to any other food or beverage that contains tryptophan. This amino acid is essential for producing serotonin—and the more of it you consume, the more serotonin your body produces!

Mind

Declining estrogen and testosterone usher in the start of the low end of your brain skills cycle that lasts through Day 2. This doesn't mean that you suddenly forget the alphabet, and long division is too complicated to even consider. But if you want an A in physics class, you're probably going to have to actually crack a book to get it.

Thinking

Concentration and the ability to absorb information isn't your problem. Making decisions might be, though. That's because plunging hormones are making your mood changes more numerous than the excuses for a celebrity meltdown. So if you're feeling a shot of noradrenaline, you'll be more critical; if you're feeling teary, you'll base your decision on whatever saves baby seals from being clubbed in the Arctic.[5] Best to put off biggies—such as which job offer to accept, whether to put all your savings into the stock market, or if you should dedicate your entire life to reviving '80s new wave fashion—till Day 6 when high estrogen and testosterone make you more confident and upbeat, which makes decision making easier and you more resolute in your choices.

Memory

You can remember most of the names, dates, and locations of items you need. But every so often your mind blanks out on facts you have down pat on high estrogen days. No biggie. Unless you've got a high-stakes game of Trivial Pursuit coming up. In which case, you might not want to bet the farm.

Verbal

Progesterone is causing a delay in word recall and verbal responses, so your end of the conversation will probably be littered with a few "umm's" and "wait-one-sec-it's-on-the-tip-of-my-tongue's."

The side of your brain highlighted today?

Right brain: Your boy toy brags that he just bought a basketball autographed by Michael Jordon for a buck online? You're like, "Sheesh, cash in a savings bond and use it to buy a clue." Your roommate told you he just answered an e-mail from a Mozambican prince who wants to pay him to store his gold bullion for him? You can't help but respond, "One hundred eighty million sperm, and you were the fastest?" Your cubicle mate tells you he just bought a Princess Diana memorial teaspoon off QVC that's guaranteed to be a collector's item? You're like, "Your village called. They want their idiot back."

Harsh not, noradrenalined one. It's not their fault they can't see the truth as clearly as you can. You've got your intuitive right brain giving you a helping hand. It's making your gut instinct a virtual Judge Judy in discerning lies from the real deal.

Creativity, writing, and introspection are also highlighted today. So you'll probably prefer blogging and updating your Friendster profile to playing Tetris and forwarding e-mail jokes as ways to goof off at work.

Romance

If you're in a relationship . . .

Does your guy have flaws? Ewww, not good for him. When mood-stabilizing serotonin is low, rip-him-a-new-one noradrenaline will be taking over. How will you know when noradrenaline has the upper hand? When your nerves feel on edge and you fly off the handle at relatively minor offenses, like your mate leaving nacho crumbs on your freshly washed Colin Farrell bedsheets . . . yet again. Sure, he may be sending you a message. But it's not a message he should be sending during hormone with-drawal. Especially if he's a bleeder.

Pity your boy. He already thinks you're an enigma wrapped in a riddle inside a potentially lethal weapon. He simply doesn't know about the power of noradrenaline, the poor dear. Help him avoid at least a few noradrena-line explosions by giving him some insider information: He can help boost your soothing serotonin with good deeds, such as giving you a reassuring hug, drawing you a hot bubble bath, or buying you the matching Colin Farrell pil-low cases.[6]

No problems in your relationship? Then do your happy dance and bake your guy a celebratory pie. It'll give you something yummy to munch on while fulfilling both pro-gesterone-induced urges to nosh and nurture.

If you're single . . .

Decreasing estrogen and testosterone have you fret-ting over your appearance and worrying about your ability to land a man. Let it get to you too much and you may resort to drastic measures—like Googling past boyfriends or trolling *www.classmates.com* for high school crushes. (The horror!)

Sex

Your libido is less noticeable than the fourth Baldwin brother. You're walking in on your guy vacuuming more often than you're thinking of sex. And when you want to get it on, withdrawing hormones are making it so much easier for the boy toy to say just the wrong thing, for instance, "Keep the light on." (As if you'd even consider baring your swollen premenstrual tummy, which you've already decided to name Harry if it's bloat and Sabrina if it's gas).

As if that wasn't enough, descending estrogen and testosterone are making you more susceptible to distractions, such as sounds[7] (your cat spitefully knocking over your "World's Greatest Cat Mom" mug), smells[8] (the cheese fries your roommate burned in the microwave, which he still hasn't cleaned up), and sights[9] (his dirty fingernails, ew).

But despite all this, you'll still feel a few pangs of lust during your day. If you want to act fast and hit the sheets before your libido goes back down or your guy has a chance to spark a noradrenaline bomb, then air out the room, slip in your favorite CD, and turn off the light to combat all distractions.

What about the quality of your orgasms—are they worth all the trouble? Well, if they could be measured on a Richter scale, they'd be about a 4.5. Not enough to flatten a whole county. But enough to shake cans off store shelves and cause some minor structural damage.

Thing is, if you want to orgasm with your man, he'll really have to be prepared for the task ahead. That's because everything is stacking up against him: Your orgasms take a few minutes longer to reach. You have less sensitivity in your nipples and clitoris. And low estrogen means lubrication is barely there. (Ouchers.)

If you want to go for it anyway, but you're out of lube or your guy is too tuckered for anything but a quickie, then take matters into your own hands. Besides the pain-squelching endorphins your orgasm produces (which translates into a brief but oh-so-welcome vacation from the swollen balloons of hell that are your breasts), orgasms also boost estrogen, which in turn improves mood and helps to relieve PMS symptoms.

Money

Decreasing estrogen and testosterone are hyping up money worries and about just how much you've got in the bank. At the same time, PMS discomfort is driving you to do some, ahem, medicinal shopping.

Want to avoid the anxiety that comes from shopping? Then buy small—a pack of gum, a loose Tic Tac perhaps. Right. That couldn't sound less appealing.

But what if you were told that curbing your spending now would be a good thing because it would help balance out all that high estrogen/high testosterone splurging from the first half of your cycle? No? Well, what if you were told that by scrimping and saving today you get those card balances down? Still no? Okay, then what if you were told . . . You know what? There's nothing else. Go ahead and shop.

Career

Worries about work are climbing. You may be concerned about meeting a deadline, wondering if you're talented enough to pull off your part of the project, or fretting over whether a pink slip is waiting for you at Human Resources.

Relax—you're job performance isn't lacking. Your optimism-inducing estrogen and security-enhancing testosterone are. Truth is, while in the right brain phase, you've got lots of creative ideas and solutions to bring to the boardroom table. So before you resign on your boss's voicemail, make a mental note to revisit these issues on Day 1 and see how differently you feel.

Energy

In recent days, progesterone had you feeling at best tranquil, at worst lethargic. But even in slow-mo you still had the endurance to make it through a whole day of work without falling asleep on your keyboard and accidentally e-mailing "kahtlakdkdalksalaaaaaaaaaaaa" to your boss. And now that estrogen and testosterone take a dive? You may want to move your keyboard out of the way when you feel a yawn coming on.

Here's a little hormonal irony for you: Even though you're feeling tired and low-key, and having difficulty staying alert during the day, once you climb into bed, your sleep isn't deep and restful. That's declining estrogen's fault. It's making you achy and your skin more sensitive, which has even the softest blankie feeling all scratchy and harsh and one itty bitty sheet wrinkle feeling like a spear being driven right into your back. Declining estrogen is also making you more sensitive to odors and sounds. This means sleeping through the smell of your roommate's burned dinner and your mate's loud snoring just got a lot more difficult.

What's more, declining estrogen is also the source of noradrenaline bursts—you know, those things that cause the temper flares every time your boyfriend says something even remotely stupid, such as, "What time will dinner be ready?" and "You look so pretty today." Well, it turns out you experience these bursts in the middle of the night, too.[10] And they're waking you up, making it difficult to fall back asleep, and keeping you from reaching a deep REM stage once you do drift off. So by the time morning comes, it's pretty much a tossup between what's got you more exhausted—a lack of pep-inducing hormones or all the nighttime tossing and turning you just did.

Luckily, there are ways to make your sleep more restful: Take ibuprofen or acetaminophen about a half hour before bedtime to reduce pain,[11] air out the room to get rid of odors,[12] mask sounds with a white noise machine or fan,[13] and try to make your bed as comfortable—and wrinkle free—as possible.

If you still wake up feeling wiped out, before you turn to your trusty friend Java Joe for a quick pick-me-up, remember that caffeine amps up PMS symptoms and boosts not-so-nice noradrenaline. That could mean lots more irritability, anxiety, and worry than even your own hormones had in store.

To keep energy up without bringing your mood down, opt instead for protein- or iron-rich snacks to pump up your energy throughout the day. And banish the guilt about taking a nap. Studies show that even a quick ten minutes of ZZZ time in the company break room can perk you up for the rest of the day.[14]

Diet

Been eating all the baddies? As progesterone declines, the intensity of the cravings you've been having for sweets, salts, carbs, fats, and comfort foods lessens just a bit. This doesn't mean a hot fudge sundae or a box of peanut brittle doesn't still have a death-grip hold over you. But you will notice that you may be able to leave the last cookie for your mate. Or at least the last half a cookie. Okay, you'll buy a whole new box for him. But you won't eat all of that box. All right, you will. But screw him. He doesn't have to deal with progesterone like you do.

Been keeping all the baddies away? Then cravings continue to be mild and infrequent for you. Boast about this too much and frustrated dieting friends may pin you down and force feed you Twinkies and Mallomars. Yuck. Not even the good stuff.

Even though progesterone begins to ebb away today, it's still making your blood sugar more sensitive. So continue to eat a snack every three to four hours to keep away the hunger crankies. And continue to include fiber in your diet to combat progesterone-induced constipation. Your bowels will thank you for it in the morning.

Look out!

You have less coordination and dexterity as balancing estrogen and testosterone decrease. What's more, alcohol is making you drunker faster from today through Day 28. Less coordination? Drunker? This definitely makes the table-top dance you'll be doing a lot more interesting.

Ouchers!

Today through Day 1, you're becoming increasingly more sensitive to anything that hurts, as plunging estrogen reduces pain-muffling endorphins. So you may want to avoid stage diving and Ultimate Fighting cage matches till estrogen rises again to a less painful level on Day 2.

Health

As estrogen and testosterone take their second plunge this cycle, they may make you vulnerable to multiple health problems:

- From Day 23 to Day 28 the abrupt change in hormone levels causes flare-ups of many chronic illnesses including asthma, depression, diabetes, digestive disorders, fibromyalgia, heart palpitations, hot flashes, multiple sclerosis, rheumatoid arthritis, and acne and other skin disorders.[15]
- Migraine alert: The sudden decline in estrogen puts you at risk of a headache or migraine, especially if you're prone to them. If you have migraine triggers—like MSG or caffeine—avoid them. If you take migraine painkillers, it's time to stock up.

Day 24

Moody Blues

Mood

Upbeat and positive? Oh sure, it has its moments. It's the only way to enjoy cotton candy. It's practically a job requirement for anyone on daytime TV. And a trip to the salon for a new 'do should never be taken when you're feeling anything other than cheerful.

But emotional and moody. Now that's got "complex, deep thinker" written all over it.

So how convenient is it that withdrawing hormones make you one complex, deep-thinking gal today? It certainly beats having to write the embarrassing, angst-filled poetry or wear the unflattering black turtleneck that would normally get you here.

Of course, even though hormone withdrawal makes you seem lots more interesting, it has its own set of drawbacks. Estrogen withdrawal, for instance, gives rise to bouts of nervousness, anxiety, teariness, and the blues. Plus, it's bringing down mood-stabilizing serotonin, which gives explosive noradrenaline a chance to bitch slap you around a little.

Sure-fire serotonin booster

Skip the Atkins Diet and load up on carbs! Turns out, carbohydrates increase serotonin! The trick is to stick to the "good carbs," which are unprocessed whole grains—such as whole wheat bread, oatmeal, and brown rice. Diving into the "bad carbs," which are processed—such as white bread, pretzels, and candy—will trigger progesterone-induced cravings. Then it's Doritos or bust!

Meanwhile, withdrawing testosterone erodes your self-confidence and has you doubting your talents, skills, and especially your appearance. Even after a tenth try at putting on your makeup, you're pretty sure Carrot Top could still beat you in a beauty contest.

And when weepy, withdrawing progesterone doesn't have your mascara running at TV commercials, it's smudging your day with crying jags over lots of other things, such as the cable going out and the unnecessary violence in Bugs Bunny cartoons.

Depending on your sensitivity to hormones and which hormone contraceptive you take, PMS symptoms will be mild and pop up only occasionally, or they could be as intense and frequent as a hangover in your junior year.

But regardless of the intensity of your PMS, withdrawal symptoms don't occur constantly. They're merely the punctuation marks in the run-on sentence that is your day. Between withdrawal symptoms, low estrogen and testosterone have you feeling thoughtful and progesterone has you feeling subdued.

When it comes to where to go and what to do today, low estrogen and testosterone are sapping your energy and decreasing your derring-do, which makes hanging out at the usual spots lots more fun than signing on for an as-yet-untried adventure. So skip the trek around Mt. Ngauruhoe or the exploration of the hanging coffins of Sagada and invite some friends over for a pizza instead.

Mind

When estrogen and testosterone rise, they improve brain skills. When estrogen and testosterone dip, well, you can see where this is headed, right?

Thinking

You know how after a few tequila shots things start to get a little fuzzy? And it's hard to concentrate? And you may not make the wisest decision? Well, today through Day 28 will be kinda like that. Some good news though— no matter how out of focus your brain gets, you won't end up with your head in the toilet.

Memory

Declining estrogen and testosterone—responsible for keeping Shoebox Greetings churning out so many belated birthday cards.

Verbal

Progesterone is placing a gap between your thoughts and your mouth, which is intermittently causing a bottleneck of stutters and false starts. The good news? Low estrogen and testosterone have you feeling less talkative, so it's a lot less noticeable than on a chattier, high estrogen day.

The side of your brain highlighted today?

Right brain: Anything you set your creative mind to today will totally rock. A stained glass doghouse. A dry macaroni replica of Michelangelo's *David*. A thong made of plastic wrap and a little bit of glitter. Anything.

Romance

If you're in a relationship . . .

He puts the empty milk carton back in the fridge. He leaves his dirty socks on the floor. He blinks. Most anything can ignite the spark that makes the boom that, invariably, he never sees coming. Have mercy on your mate. For he must now walk through the minefield that is your noradrenaline.

Is your guy on his best behavior and dutifully leaving offerings of junk food and chick-flick DVDs at the goddess of noradrenaline's perfectly pedicured feet? Then progesterone will have you repaying him with nurturing kindness. You'll feel like brewing him a cup of delicious, hot cocoa, fluffing up his pillow, and putting nonslip stickers in the bathtub so he doesn't fall and hurt himself doing the shower karaoke he doesn't know you're peeking in on.

If you're single . . .

With your right brain introspection high and confidence in your appearance low, it's got you feeling doubtful about current prospects and wondering if you're still hot enough to attract a new guy. The result? You may be tempted to call up lads you kicked to the curb long ago. Want to resist the temptation? Taking a moment to remember why your relationship didn't work out the first time may help. Looking at the ad he put up on Yahoo! Personals one day after your break up may help more.

Sex

Your emotions are a kaleidoscope of change. Absolutely. Noradrenaline is hiding behind every corner. No doubt. And everyone whose libido is lower than the introductory rate on a preapproved credit card, take one step forward.

Not so fast, Day 24 Girl. In an unexpected twist, your libido shoots up today and keeps increasing all the way through Day 28. Even as sex-craving testosterone continues to take a serious dive? Yes. Even as libido-dampening progesterone is still on the scene? Yes, yes.

Perplexed? So are researchers who believe that the unplanned passion isn't due to your hormones at all. Instead, they speculate it's probably a side effect of your endometrium lining.[1] As it gets thicker, it's bringing more blood flow to your vaginal area, which the researchers suspect is inadvertently stimulating you.[2]

In addition to a revved up sex drive, orgasms are also becoming more intense. The reasons behind it are still murky. But, once you reach the teeth-clenching, powerful climaxes your body's giving you, will you really care why?

Thing is, getting to that orgasmic point might take some work. That's because low estrogen and testosterone are making it easy to lose your focus. One sec you're thinking about the hunky guy in bed with you—or the hunky guy of your fantasies that's in bed with you and your vibrator. The next thing you know, the scent of your aromatherapy candle on the nightstand reminds you of your new dishwashing liquid, which reminds you of the dishes in the sink, which reminds you that your inconsiderate roommate always leaves his plates for you and this time you're going to leave them for him. By the time your thoughts have made the return trip to your quest for an orgasm, you find that your boy's already finished or your batteries are kaput.

One other thing to be aware of today is that you're not producing enough lubrication to last you through a marathon sex session. That's low estrogen's fault. And it gets even lower as the rest of your cycle goes on. So be sure to stock up on some KY before you climb into bed with a partner or you'll be rubbed too raw to enjoy the sexual pleasure that Days 25, 26, 27, and 28 have in store.

Money

No doubt about it—PMS sucks. Your breasts are so sore that simply breathing makes them hurt. You've got a pick-a-mood-any-mood thing going on. And the bloat, well, let's just say it feels like a water balloon has a less fluid-to-tissue ratio than you.

So what's all this possibly have to do with shopping? Try everything. Turns out, shopping increases endorphins, which help relieve PMS symptoms by easing pain and elevating mood. Not only that, but the walking that you're doing as you shop can even alleviate some of that water retention that's causing bloat and sore breasts!

Just one word of warning: Don't spend more than you can handle. Declining estrogen and testosterone are pumping up worry over finances, which means that the uplifting mood shopping gave you can be instantly transformed into a blue funk once you get home and realize you'll be paying off your student loans before your MasterCard bill.

Career

Concerns about stability at work are on your mind. You want to know that your job is secure, that you've got a future there, that you're meeting your company's expectations. Basically, withdrawing estrogen and testosterone want your boss to send you a Mylar balloon bouquet with

"Good Job! Your 401(k) is so not going to be blown on private planes and weeklong parties!" emblazoned on them.

The truth about the pension is anybody's guess. But no Mylar nosegay is needed to reassure you about your work skills. With right brain problem-solving and brainstorming abilities highlighted, you can come up with surprising solutions and creative proposals for practically any situation. And with your writing ability stronger, you can type yourself a note to remind yourself of just how talented you are when low estrogen and testosterone have you forgetting. And another note to remind yourself to inquire about the status of that 401(k).

Energy

You're tired, sluggish, and longing for a nap as estrogen and testosterone continue their downward slide and take your energy and endurance with them. And, adding drowsiness to exhaustion, sleep is less restorative as noradrenaline bursts and increased sensitivity to pain, odors, and noise wake you up in the middle of the night.

Want to sleep more soundly tonight? Taking a pain reliever a half hour before turning in, removing smelly items, and masking sounds with a white noise machine or fan can help. Surprisingly, drinking till you pass out won't. Turns out that alcohol may get you to sleep quicker, but it also makes sleep even more interrupted than before. And sleeping pills? Well, they may work temporarily, but they also affect your short-term memory, something that's already taking a beating during this low hormone stage.[3] If you really want to try a tincture that will get you to sleep more soundly, you're better off sticking to tried-and-true favorites such as chamomile tea or warm milk.[4]

Looking for more zest during your daytime hours? Avoid caffeine, since it can worsen PMS symptoms and make noradrenaline bursts more frequent. Instead, opt for healthier alternatives. such as popping an iron supplement or eating foods rich in energizing iron, such as steak, chicken, wheat germ, or spinach.

Diet

Got a yen for sweets, salts, carbs, fats, and comfort foods? Yes? Busted! You've been eating junk food all along, haven't you? No biggie. But it won't help the food cravings any.

Don't have any cravings for sweets, salt, carbs, fats, and comfort foods? Then you've probably been avoiding them this whole time. Either that or you've never had sweets, salts, carbs, fats, or comfort foods and you don't realize what you're missing. If you want to remain blissfully ignorant and craving free, then never step foot in Cinnabon in your life.

Even though progesterone continues to decrease, keep adding fiber to your diet to prevent constipation. And continue eating every three to four hours to keep the hunger grumblies away.

An Emotional Wild Card

Mood

Another day, another ride on the moody merry-go-round. One minute you're breaking out into spontaneous sobbing while putting sprinkles on cupcakes. The next minute you're feeling as on-edge as a billionaire CEO facing a Senate investigation. Another minute later, you're so down on yourself, you figure a reality show contestant could outperform you. One minute after that, you're so sad, you're pretty sure if you hear about one more endangered animal being forced out of its home because of illegal logging or if the vending machine in the employee lounge breaks down just one more time, you're seriously going to need a Prozac smoothie. But then, a minute later, you're feeling all right again—happy even. At least for another minute.

Rest assured—it's merely withdrawing estrogen, testosterone, and progesterone. They're like three hands battling to control the sock puppet of your emotions. You'll know which one has taken over by their trademark symptoms: Withdrawing estrogen is the one making you anxious and sad; withdrawing testosterone is the one sapping you of your confidence and security; and withdrawing progesterone is the one making you go through Kleenex with the speed of a twelve-year-old stuffing her bra.

On top of all these mood changes, you also have jump-you-from-behind noradrenaline filling you with rage at every bank error, stubbed toe, and looped on-hold recording that assures you "an operator will be with you momentarily."

Depending on your hormone sensitivity and what kind of hormone contraceptives you use, you'll experience many or just a few of these rapid-fire mood changes and noradrenaline rushes throughout your day.

Between withdrawal symptoms, low estrogen and testosterone have you feeling thoughtful and introspective, and progesterone has you feeling low-key. Adventure, thrills, and risks are probably as appealing to you today as fat-free potato chips. Instead, you'll be happiest when you're with close friends in familiar places.

Sure-fire serotonin booster

Turn on another lamp! Studies show exposure to more light increases serotonin!

Mind

As estrogen and testosterone decline, they continue to take the shine off your brain skills. But your creative right brain gets all evil genius to make up for it.

Thinking

It's not as though you're at blank-stare levels today. But you may find it more difficult to keep your attention while performing certain boring tasks, such as reading an instruction manual or watching whatever Hilary Duff movie is on TV.

When it comes to making decisions, your mood is still subject to change without notice from declining estrogen and testosterone. So put off biggies that can't be reversed—such as whether to sink all your savings into your friend's start-up company or sell the house and tool around the country in an Airstream—till Day 6 when estrogen and testosterone get your decision-making skills rising to more resolute levels.

Memory

No doubt you'll be able to remember the essential stuff—where you parked the car or what street your home's on. But the name of the new guy who says hi every time he passes the desk? A mystery.

Verbal

Progesterone is throwing roadblocks into your sentences, making your speech stop and start more frequently than rush-hour traffic. And declining estrogen and testosterone are no help as they make remembering the right word so much harder. This combination has you feeling like there is a four-car pile-up on the tip of your tongue.

The side of your brain highlighted today?

Right brain: Creative power—while in the right brain phase you've got lots of it. Depending on your mood, you can use it for good—crafting a handy potholder for your best friend; or for evil—carving butter to look like a bar of soap and leaving it in your clean-freak-of-a-roommate's bath caddy.

If you choose the latter and can't manage to stifle the laughter and talk your way out of your obvious guilt, then do the right thing—sit down at the computer and write a lovely haiku explaining exactly what drove you to do what you did. (You de-lint carpet / Dust your toothbrush and pet cat / Stop, anal dirt thief!) No doubt she'll be moving out next month, but at least you won't have missed a chance to show off your stellar right brain writing skills.

After you've finished placing your ad on Craigslist for a new roommate, your introspective side has you mulling over more serious issues in your life, such as what to do about the ex who won't stop calling, how to get your boss to notice your hard work, and which three-piece rims you should go with when you pimp your ride.

Romance

If you're in a relationship . . .

Did he forget your half-year anniversary? Is he bogarting the remote and refusing to stay on one channel longer than a nanosecond? Has he still not fixed that hole in the wall he made while trying to slam-dunk the frozen Thanksgiving turkey into his indoor basketball hoop? On high estrogen days you'd probably let it all slide. Today? He'd better have two tickets for a cruise to the French Riviera or a lifetime membership to Chocolates R Us handy to appease the goddess of noradrenaline, whom he has angered.

Is all well in the land of love? Gals with imperfect mates hate you, you know that, right? But you can redeem yourself by sharing some of those homemade cookies and cakes that nurturing progesterone has you baking for your perfecter than perfect man.

If you're single . . .

Like a dysfunctional family, decreasing estrogen and testosterone are trying to undermine your confidence and have you thinking you're not as smart or pretty as all the other girls. But a rising libido is urging you to go catch yourself a stud anyway. The result? You may find yourself more willing to accept an old lover's last-minute booty call because you can avoid that whole first-time-naked thing. Or you may lower your high-estrogen-day standards and end up slumming it with a guy who thinks he's showing off by spelling his name in the snow with pee.

By Day 1, you know you deserve better than that. So if oxytocin from sex hasn't already bonded you to the guy you're settling for today, he'll likely be toast by the start of your next cycle.

Sex

Your libido started coming to life yesterday. Okay, it probably started coming to life the first time Luke Perry and his gravity-defying hair swaggered into the malt shop on 90210. But let's skip ahead and start with Day 24, when your sex drive began increasing once again after a brief progesterone-induced guy-atus. Researchers speculate that this libido boost is caused by your thickening endometrium, since it's bringing more blood flow to your nether regions, which makes you aroused more easily. If that's the case, then you'll feel even more moments of sexual arousal since your endometrium gets thicker today, bringing even more blood flow to your special place.

What researchers haven't figured out yet is why orgasms seem to also get increasingly intense as Day 28 closes in. Could it be a gift from your biology for having to put up with PMS? Perhaps a side effect of eating two dozen Ring Dings and a half a box of Hostess Ho Hos? It's all still a mystery. Luckily, that mystery needn't be solved in order for you to enjoy the climaxes that feel as amazing as on any high testosterone day. And if you remember nothing else from Days 1 through 13, it's definitely the felt-all-over explosions that were your orgasms.

Now here's the tricky part. Your orgasms may feel like the ones you have on high testosterone days. But getting there? Um, not so much. Decreasing estrogen and testosterone make you more easily distracted by sights, sounds, and smells, as well as issues that your right brain has been churning up these past few days. And let's face it, stewing about your lad's insensitivity while he's pumping away is no direct route to climax.

What's more, your body is producing only minimal amounts of lubricant while estrogen is low. So don't be afraid to pull out the store-bought kind. That is, unless raw, itchy thrust-burn is what gets you through your day.

On top of it all, it's taking a few minutes longer than on a high testosterone day to orgasm. So if your guy doesn't have the endurance to wait it out, you could be heading for the toy box after he leaves. Or you could opt to skip the boy and head straight for the toy instead. After all, whether they're self-induced or sex-induced, orgasms flood your system with pain-blunting endorphins and boost estrogen, which in turn elevates mood and helps ease PMS symptoms. And, really, doesn't that make the few extra minutes going for your O worth it?

Money

Money worries are high as estrogen and testosterone decrease. Yet impulsively spending on stuff you so don't need seems to make the pain of PMS so much less.

Oh, which influence to follow? Which influence to follow?

No, this book can't make up your mind for you. But it *can* tell you that shopping releases endorphins, which lift your mood and help alleviate premenstrual pain that's causing aches, pains, and sensitive skin. And this book *can* inform you that even buying something small—say, a new lipstick or CD—is enough to trigger these brain chemicals. And it *can* suggest that if you do go on a buying bender, you could justify your purchases by saying that shopping could technically qualify as a sort of PMS therapy. You know, just in case any low estrogen and testosterone guilties show up after the sale. But this book definitely *cannot* make up your mind for you.

Career

As estrogen and testosterone continue to decrease during your right brain introspective phase, you've got concerns about the security of your job, and every once in a while you may wonder if this is really the right place for you.

If you do decide to stay put at your current place of employment, then you're most impressive when using your right brain talents to work on creative projects and brainstorm inventive solutions. During your right brain phase, you also excel at writing, which can help you get around the lack of verbal fluency you've been experiencing as your brain skills move to the low end of their cycles. Or it could help you craft really funny messages for your game of interoffice text message tag.

Energy

You remember all those high-energy activities you were doing on Day 13? The thought of doing them today won't even cross your mind. And if it does, then you're either drinking lots of caffeine (bad idea since it makes PMS so much worse), you're required to do them for your job (hey, you could be a performer for Cirque de Soleil), or you need an intervention for your crank habit (or Red Bull addiction—sometimes it's so hard to tell the difference).

All other gals, you'll feel like taking it leisurely today as estrogen and testosterone continue to plunge and take your energy and endurance down with them.

Having trouble sleeping through the aches and pains, odors, noise, and noradrenaline bursts? The aches and pains can be fought off with a pain reliever about thirty minutes before you turn in. The odors can be squashed by airing out your bedroom and not letting your boyfriend order the bean burritos. And sleep-busting sounds can be drowned out with a white noise machine or air conditioner.

Now the noradrenaline bursts, you're pretty much on your own there. But if you've been avoiding caffeine, then at least you won't be increasing the number of sleep-interrupting bursts you have.

In place of PMS-intensifying caffeine, boost your zip and stamina during the day by snacking on peanuts, a spinach salad, a burger, or any other food loaded in energizing protein and iron.

Diet

Been giving in to your cravings for sweets, salts, carbs, fats, and comfort foods since Day 14 began? Then why stop now? You're smack in the middle of PMS and comfort food can actually help improve your mood.[1]

Haven't touched the baddies yet? Then you may be missing out on the mood-elevating effects of nutritional no-nos, but at least you don't have to deal with the progesterone-induced cravings that seem to jump you from behind at every convenience store and supermarket.

Keep the fiber coming and continue to nosh your way through the day to prevent the hunger crankies from taking over.

Health

The decline of estrogen signals the rise in the potential for health problems:

- Asthma alert: 75 percent of asthma attacks occur either during or shortly before menstruation.[2]
- Migraine alert: Plunging estrogen makes today through Day 3 a high-risk day for menstrual migraine. So avoid migraine triggers, such as caffeine, citrus fruits, salt, and food preservatives.

The Good, the Bad, the Sexy

Mood

Blue moods, crying jags, noradrenaline bursts. Hormone withdrawal can be a total drag. Especially if you're hormone sensitive. Then decreasing estrogen, testosterone, and progesterone have you experiencing these here-one-minute-gone-the-next emotions with irritating frequency and intensity.

Take hormone contraceptives? Then you've probably run out of hormones by now. In which case, PMS is finally hitting you full force. Try to avoid too much complaining around girlfriends who've been putting up with full-throttle PMS since Day 23. They may be tempted to replace your contraceptives with Pez to show you what you've been missing.

But regardless of your hormone sensitivity, or whether your hormones just ran out, withdrawal symptoms don't last all day without a break. In between, low estrogen and testosterone are making your mood mellow and introspective. And progesterone continues to keep you feeling tranquil. This laidback state may make it difficult to

235

feel inspired or motivated. Unless, of course, cookies are somehow involved. In which case, you are *so* there.

Falling testosterone has you shying away from daring, untried adventures. And decreasing estrogen has your emotions a tad sensitive to the people and events around you. So you're happiest when things are predictable and familiar. Which means activities such as mosh pitting, stage diving, and midnight madness bowling are out. Ditto for that silk flowers convention that always draws a wild crowd.

You're happiest sticking to activities that are nice and slow. Things your grandma would like, such as meeting up with close friends at a quaint tearoom or getting a steamy DVD for softcore porn flick night. What? As if Grandma never watched softcore porn? Puhleeze. Don't be so naive . . .

Sure-fire serotonin booster

Ask your honey for a massage. Even if he wimps out and gives you a quickie, studies show that all it takes is a few minutes to elevate serotonin!

Mind

Estrogen and testosterone are taking a dive and they're taking your brain skills down with them. Luckily, you've still got creativity to show off.

Thinking

Losing your focus every so often? Most likely. Finding it hard to absorb new info? At least a little. Decisions harder to make than a soufflé at a *Lord of the Dance* rehearsal? You'll get no argument here.

Memory

Right about now you're probably wondering if that Ginko biloba stuff really works. It might. But a PDA works a whole lot better.

Verbal

The halting, stuttering effect seems to be dwindling as progesterone decreases. But it's so difficult to notice an improvement when plunging estrogen and testosterone continue to make recalling the right word and talking fluently so much harder.

The side of your brain highlighted today?

Right brain: What declining estrogen and testosterone are taking away in thinking, memory, and verbal ability, they're making up for in creativity. Does a boring coworker need your help perking up the "interests" line on her resumé? Without batting an eye, you're scribbling down hobbies that make her seem more fascinating than Mark Walhberg's third nipple. Is your marketing executive boyfriend wracking his brain for a cool new ad campaign for his client? You assure him you'll come up with an idea worthy of a Clio Award . . . right after you're done designing the fountain you're going to install in the backyard and putting the finishing touches on your latest Rice-A-Roni sculpture.

When not pursuing creative plans, your thoughts turn inward. You're thinking about goals you set aside but still want to pursue (like attending acting classes or joining the space program) and issues that need to be resolved (such as breaking it to your hairdresser than you've found someone new, someone Sassoon-trained and who does Japanese straightening—and you're very happy together).

Romance

If you're in a relationship . . .

He leaves the seat up in the middle of the night. He eats the last Krispy Kreme. He asks you if the guys can come over to watch the game *after* he's already invited them. All will pretty much answer the question about that whole noradrenaline thingy.

Is your guy on his best behavior? Nice training. Reward both of you for a job well done by using your progesterone-induced nurturing feelings to whip up a yummy home-cooked meal or dial up your favorite takeout restaurant.

If you're single . . .

Declining estrogen and testosterone have you doubting your appearance. But a rising libido has you interested in flirting and finding a sex partner. The result: You may find yourself attracted to more "sure bets." You know, men you probably wouldn't give a second glance to on higher estrogen days, for instance, that guy who keeps flashing his gold Faux-lex watch or the dude who thinks his beer-bong hat can accessorize any outfit.

You may also feel an urge to try out image enhancers that you would have flat-out rejected on rising estrogen and testosterone days. Such as? Such as a chemical peel, nose job, or Botox for your sweat pores. Put off doing anything too painful and by Day 1, when confidence in your appearance rises along with your estrogen and testosterone levels, you'll probably feel like you dodged a bullet. Or at least six to eight weeks of painful recovery.

Sex

Just when you thought plunging hormones were taking the last of your stable mood, brain skills, and energy with them, your body pops up with some lovely parting gifts: the libido of a forty-year-old virgin and orgasms that are so powerful you're pretty sure that if harnessed properly they could provide an alternative energy source for an entire city block.

The reason for the carnal upswell? That uterine wall thickening and bringing more bloodflow to your vagina. And when there's more bloodflow, you become more aroused. It's the same thing that happens when testosterone rises or when you think naughty thoughts. *Very* naughty thoughts.

Give in to the urge to go for the O either with your boy or alone and you'll help relieve PMS by boosting endorphins, which temporarily block pain, oxytocin, which helps you sleep more soundly, and estrogen, which improves your mood.

Need another reason to go for the O? Really? Then you probably have never experienced one. In which case, get thee to Amazon.com for a how-to book. Buy a toy from an online sex aid store run by sex therapists such as *www.libida.com* or *www.myPleasure.com*. Head to an erotic bookshop or video store to stock up on orgasm-inducing sexual fantasies. Call a sex therapist for intensive instruction. Or simply spend all your free time masturbating till you get it right.

Money

The human body—it seems as if it's always telling you how to make it feel better. You feel thirsty; your body tells you to take a drink. You feel hungry; your body tells you to eat some food. Your endorphins plunge; your body tells you shopping will bring instant relief.

And it will. That is, till decreasing estrogen and testosterone get wind of your splurging. Then it's all, "Your bank balance is low" this and "You're going to be in debt for the rest of your life" that. Bitch. Bitch. Bitch. Don't these hormones have moods to change or noradrenaline fuses to light? Yes. But when they're on the decline, as they are today, they'll still make time to stick you with guilt and worry over purchases, too.

Career

Sure, every job has its downsides. But they're just so much easier to see when estrogen and testosterone are declining. The boss's e-mailed jokes seem so much lamer, the pay seems so much crappier, and the smell drifting from the kitchen fridge seems more and more nauseating by the minute.

But if you can get past all that, then you'll be contributing creative ideas, brainstorming inventive solutions, writing eloquent reports, and sending polite **LOLs** to your boss's many lame joke-filled e-mails with ease.

Energy

Decreasing estrogen and testosterone—they're trying to make you too fatigued to do anything fun, such as drinks after work with the gals, a late-night party, or your weekly extreme yoga class. They'd rather you just stay home and become one with the couch cushions.

Unfortunately, getting deep, energy-restoring sleep is still a difficult task as you continue to experience sleepus interruptus from declining estrogen. Keep taking a pain reliever before bedtime, airing out the room, and putting on a noise-masking fan. And if a noradrenaline burst wakes you and you have trouble getting back to sleep, drinking a cup of soothing chamomile tea or warm milk may help.

If you're looking to boost daytime pep, skip the caffeine. Quick energy rushes make PMS much more of a cranky experience. Instead, go for iron- and protein-rich snacks, which give you a steadier supply of energy and don't exacerbate PMS symptoms.

Diet

If you've been giving in to cravings for sweets, salts, carbs, fats, and comfort foods, the cravings decrease as progesterone decreases. And on Day 1, you begin to eat 12 percent less. So you may as well use these last cravings to polish off the rest of the doughnuts and chips.

If you've been cutting out the yummy stuff all along, then cravings have been low during this entire progesterone-dominated phase. Keep it to yourself and your girlfriends might not inject Crisco into your tofu.

Continue including fiber in your diet and eating a snack every three to four hours. Even though progesterone is getting lower by the day, it's still enough to affect your digestion and blood sugar.

Day 27

A Hut of One's Own

Mood

Old school: Women check into the village menstrual hut and chill out with other menstruating gals.[1]

New school: Women hibernate on the living room couch and conference call their girlfriends.

Old school: While holed up in the menstrual hut, women experiment with various poultices to chase away cramps, try out the latest in wild berry lip stain, and entertain each other with colorful stories about which of their various gods recently smote whom, who's the hunkiest warrior in the tribe, and if they believe all the rumors about a swarm of locusts coming to eat the crops.

New school: While holed up on the couch, women pop Advil before their period begins to prevent cramps from starting, test out the latest shade of lip gloss from Maybelline, and order up a chick-flick on Pay-Per-View.

Day 15   Day 16   Day 17   Day 18   Day 19   Day 20   Day 21

Old school: Women wait till bleeding starts to enter the menstrual hut and begin the pampering process.

New school: You don't need to bleed to prove you deserve a time-out and a little pampering. By Day 27, descending hormones are already sending you the message to kick back, relax, and take it easy.[2] And that message is being sent in so many ways:

- You're quieter, slower, and your skin is more sensitive to pain on a day when your coordination is lowest and you're banging into more table corners, doorways, and chairs.

- You've still got that whole emotional Ferris wheel thing going on where you're cycling through bouts of the blues, anxiety, insecurity, and teariness. And noradrenaline bursts continue to pounce on every wrong answer your guy gives to the "Does this make me look fat?" question.

- And, when you're not having mood swings or noradrenaline temper flares, your energy level is so low and your breasts so sore, that the last place you'd want to be is competing in the Iron Man or high-heeling it through a giant elbowed amoeba of dancers on your way to the lone empty barstool on the other side of the club that will be taken by the time you reach it anyway.

So, go ahead and give in to the urge to pamper yourself. It raises serotonin and endorphin levels, which help lift your mood and alleviate pain. And it may be the last rest stop you get before Day 4 when the all-night blowouts start up once again.

Sure-fire serotonin booster

Take a warm shower! Research shows that just a few minutes is all that's needed to elevate serotonin!

Mind

Estrogen and testosterone are just one day away from bottoming out completely. Which means your brain skills can't be far behind.

Thinking
You're distracted by the little things—ringing phones, beeping IMs, e-mails that seem to come in endless succession from people who couldn't reach you on the phone or by IM. It's taking you a little longer to absorb new information. And coming to a decision about even minor issues—such as which color mascara to wear or what emoticon to use—seem to take forever.

Memory
You have many skills and talents. Remembering where you put your keys simply isn't one of them. Well, at least not till memory-enhancing estrogen starts to rise again.

Verbal

So yeah, it was a little embarrassing when you told your boss, "The information was erogenous" when you meant to say "erroneous." And no doubt it's frustrating when you can't recall the same SAT words that, less than two weeks ago, you were spitting out like a fat-free bran muffin you thought was your usual double chocolate. But look at it this way—if you were verbally fluent all month long, your boss would give you all the boring tasks, such as presenting the reports at meetings or recording the messages on the voicemail system.

The side of your brain highlighted today?

Right brain: Your creativity is high. And that's akin to having a lawyer on retainer. Every time you have a problem, you can simply sic it on the problem to make it go away. For instance? Well, say you want a job that doesn't make you fantasize every day about ripping off your boss's skin with the adhesive tape on FedEx packages? You might use your creative streak to make a list of employment possibilities that will guarantee you'll like who you're working for, like becoming Johnny Depp's personal assistant or the president of your own company. Perhaps you need a new apartment that smells a little less like decaying rat? You could come up with ingenious ways to find out about openings, such as asking friends about empty apartments in their buildings or cruising the obits for recent vacancies. Are you looking for a boyfriend who believes high heels, bikini waxing, and Wonderbras were invented by misogynists who are afraid of women's innate beauty and power?

Then you may come up with imaginative ways to find him, such as signing up for a women's studies class or crashing an Alan Alda fan club meeting.

When not busy using your imagination to get out of a jam, your thoughts turn inward. You're mulling over lots of life issues, such as goals you want to achieve, your latest theories of the universe, and what gives Cheez Wiz its surprisingly long shelf life.

Romance

If you're in a relationship . . .

Your guy flawed? Declining estrogen and testosterone continue to have you seeing his foibles. But you're likely too tired to fight about whatever dunderhead thing he's done now.

Is your guy free of flaws? Progesterone is at near nonexistent levels. So his perfection may be worth praising, but nurturing time for him is over. Now it's his turn to nurture you. Which means whatever you two do together, it'll likely be at home, involving him cooking for you (or dialing up takeout), and if he's as perfect as you say, you'll have total control over the remote.

If you're single . . .

Your sex drive is high, but your desire to go out there and find a partner is low. However, if you happen to be in a situation where a man is readily available—the grocery store, copy room, parking lot—you might go for it.

Here's something you may want to keep in mind before you break out the condoms for Mr. Parking Lot Attendant. Estrogen and testosterone are making you self-conscious about your appearance. So you may be tempted to go for a guy who doesn't meet your usual high-estrogen-day standards. You know you shouldn't. You know on a higher estrogen day you wouldn't. But, hey, sex is still sex. So, it happens. No biggie, as long as oxytocin produced by intercourse doesn't instantly bond you to him. Because by the time you realize you could've done better, something may have already tied you two together forever, say, a baby or, gosh forbid, a jointly purchased timeshare.

Sex

As your uterine lining gets thicker and thicker, you become more and more easily aroused, your libido gets stronger, and the intensity of your orgasms increases. So the only news you need to know today is: Your uterine lining is getting way thicker. You may want to get the boy a B_{12} shot or head out for a fresh pack of batteries right about now.

Money

Things really take a turn for the purse today. After five days of PMS with one more to go, you're ready to indulge your every impulse-buying whim.

And what do declining estrogen and testosterone

have to say about all the freewheeling spending going on? Frankly, at this point you likely don't care. And if they do threaten to make you feel worried or anxious over your finances, you'll probably just tell them to eff off. You're buying the $150 pashmina scarf anyway.

Career

Problems at work are easier to see as estrogen and testosterone continue to decrease. But with your energy low, you're less likely to react by tipping over your faux-wood desk and recruiting the other employees to stage a mass walk-out, and more likely to simply scratch "work sux" into the bathroom stall and pocket some office creamer.

If you happen to actually like your job (hey, you could be a billionaire real-estate magnate or an official taster for Godiva) or can deal with its problems for at least one more pay period, the tasks you'll excel at today are those that use your creativity, problem-solving skills, and writing ability, which are all heightened during this right brain phase.

Energy

Right about now, you may be envying the energy level of the two-toed sloth. Especially if you're not loading up on energizing foods rich in iron and protein. And if you aren't, then declining estrogen and testosterone are really kicking the pep out of you.

Day 15 Day 16 Day 17 Day 18 Day 19 Day 20 Day 21

For a deeper night's sleep, take a pain reliever thirty minutes before bedtime, air out the room, and mask noise. And if a noradrenaline burst wakes you, resist the urge to watch TV, which can arouse your emotions and end up keeping you up even longer.[3] Instead, do something low-key that doesn't engage your mind, knitting, for example. Or reading *The Enquirer*.

Diet

Progesterone is just one day away from bottoming out. If you've been indulging in all the baddies, this means your cravings are getting lower and lower, too. Oh, you're still noshing here and there. But you're no longer junk food's bitch.

But whether you've given in to temptation or stood your nutritional ground, progesterone may be down, but it's not out. So add fiber to your diet to combat progesterone-induced constipation and snack every three to four hours to ward off the hunger meanies.

Cramp alert!

Start taking ibuprofen (such as Advil or Motrin) today. This will prevent the development of prostaglandins—hormonelike substances that cause the inflammation and pain of menstrual cramps. The result? On Day 1, you'll experience fewer cramps— or even prevent cramps from occurring altogether![4]

Dude, Where's My Hormones?

Mood

Estrogen, testosterone, and progesterone are all plummeting to the bottom of the chart today and, like accomplices looking for a plea deal, they're taking you down with them.[1]

This means you're putting up with one more day of withdrawal symptoms—anxiety, weepiness, blue moods, insecurity, and gets-in-its-last-licks-while-it-still-can noradrenaline. Depending on your hormone sensitivity, these rounds could be frequent and land knockout punches or few and far between, landing only pillow-soft blows.

With so much low-hormone discomfort, which has seemed to last for, like, ever, and extra sensitivity to the stinky, noisy, irritating world around you, your inner Naomi Campbell will probably be strutting out today. You want things your way—and if they don't go your way, you may resort to a little foot stomping, pouty whimpering, or whining in that voice that makes a Yoko Ono CD sound soothing.

Who can blame you, though? You're putting up with lots—aches, pains, low energy, moodiness, low coordination that has you knocking into every doorframe and end table in sight. If only PMS came with a cast and crutches like a broken leg. Then everyone would know just by looking that you're not feeling your best so you deserve the royal treatment. It would certainly save you the trouble of having to come right out and tell them.

Sure-fire serotonin booster

Eat only the frosting on the cake. Soak for hours in a luxurious bubble bath while ignoring all pleas from pee-pee dancing roommates. Or dare to take control of the remote and force the entire household to watch the Oxygen channel. Giving yourself permission to indulge in your guiltiest of pleasures raises serotonin and endorphin levels, which help lift your mood and alleviate pain!

Mind

Just because it feels as if your brain skills are all on par with the mental abilities of a Jell-O fruit mold doesn't mean they really are. They're simply reaching the low end of your cycle today. Which is still better than most men any day.

Thinking

This would normally be the place that would explain what fuzzy thinking is. But you've probably lost your place or gotten distracted and moved on to the next section already.

Memory

You know how that stoner guy you knew from college had no short-term memory and couldn't even remember the last thing he said? Well, your brain is going to that very special place today.

Verbal

At times—okay at many, many times—it feels as if you've got a log jam of words trying to get through the pretzel that is now your tongue. So maybe it's a good thing you're feeling about as talkative as Teller right now.

The side of your brain highlighted today?

Right brain: If it seems as if you're getting hit with a flash of inspiration with every passing moment, it's because you're deep in your creative right brain. And that makes coming up with brilliant ideas second only to breathing. Or using sticky notes to de-lint.

The lower your estrogen and testosterone go, the more your right brain skills peak. Seem like a high price to pay for some introspection, intuition, and imagination? Then beat descending hormones at their own game by using these maxed out skills to combat their withdrawal symptoms. How so? Since having fun bumps up feel-good brain chemicals like serotonin, dopamine, and endorphins, get creative about it. Double the chocolate in your hot cocoa. Warm up your undies in the dryer before putting them on. Or call a telemarketing center and keep them on the line for twenty minutes while you convince them to send *you* money.

Romance

If you're in a relationship . . .

Fantasy: Your guy, taking his cue from the wonderful nurturing you gave him on high progesterone days, is now eager to bestow loving care all over you. He's brewing you tea, bringing you pizza, and gently massaging your feet.

Reality: Your guy, who was either oblivious to all your loving care or has recently been overcome with amnesia, is looking over at you and your peeved expression wondering, "What's her problem?"

How to make your Fantasy his Reality: Come right out and ask him for what you want. Fact is, your boy would be delighted to be your fantasy nurturer.[2] He just needs you to give him clear and specific directions.[3]

Unfortunately, with bottoming out estrogen and testosterone decreasing your assertiveness, making this kind of direct request is more difficult. Instead, you're more likely to try gentle hints, meaningful glances, and sending telepathic messages. But you may as well be trying to communicate with a potato chip. Men's minds simply aren't wired to pick up on the kind of subtle language that women's are.

If you can summon the nerve to be direct, then simply explain to him exactly what you need and why. For instance, tell him you need him to run out and get you a malted milkshake because it will boost your endorphins and make you happier. Tell him you need him to give you a gentle massage because it will boost serotonin and make you happier. And tell him you need him to cancel his game-date with the guys because he has to be on hand in case you think of anything else he can do to make you happier.

If you're single . . .

Your libido may be high, but with your estrogen and testosterone so low, your heart's just not in the game. You've got zero energy, your self-confidence is at will-date-ex-boy-band-members levels and your breasts hurt so much you've got police tape set up in a ten-foot perimeter around them.

$\int e\, x$

Today, congestion in your uterus is the highest it's going to get before your period. And since congestion has been what's causing that spike in libido and the intense orgasms in recent days, you can pretty much guess what this means. That you'll be leaving your bed only for pee breaks or in case of fire? Exactly.

There's a hitch, though. Your breasts are sore, and with estrogen near bottom levels even the tenderest touch feels like a bat whacking a piñata. What to do? Well, you can either take matters into your own gentle hands or tell your guy to proceed with caution. And to forget about going near second base altogether.

Another problem you'll have to contend with is that you continue to be easily distracted as estrogen and testosterone descend. But you can keep distractions to a minimum by simply getting rid of all the things that make you lose your focus. For instance, if the smell from your guy's day-old workout shorts rankles your low estrogen nose, throw the shorts in the hamper and air out the room. If low estrogen and testosterone continue to make you worry about your body, dim the lights. If the couple next door is fighting loudly again, put on a CD to drown them out. And if there's a chance that your guy will say anything that will have your thoughts spinning off in any other direction than the sex you're having, tell him there's a pizza in it for him afterwards if he keeps his mouth shut.

One other thing: Low estrogen means that lubrication is slow and not so plentiful. So if you see that you're headed for a marathon session, break out the bottle of personal lubricant before any serious chafing stops you from reaching what is sure to be a very worth-a-marathon-session orgasm.

Money

On the last day of your cycle, you may not have the energy to vacuum, clean out your purse, or organize the DVDs. But you will have enough pep to leaf through catalogs, surf store Web sites, and call up the Home Shopping Network with the greatest of ease.

And will decreasing estrogen and testosterone be guilting you out over all the impulse buys? Oh, they'll try.

But once you recall that it was those two who helped get you into this PMS fix to begin with, it'll be so much easier to blow them off.

Career

If your job needs you to come up with a creative idea, brainstorm an inventive solution, or write an award-winning proposal, you are so there. That's because while in your right brain phase, these skills come far easier.

If your job requires you to cheerlead, roller derby, or pull an airplane with your teeth, you may want to call in sick. With estrogen and testosterone so low, your energy is taking a serious nosedive.

If your job needs you to pledge your undying devotion and loyalty, you may want to hold off till tomorrow. That's when rising estrogen and testosterone will have you feeling all warm and gooey about your employer again. But today? Um, not so much.

Look out!

Put away the pompoms and hang up the flaming batons. With estrogen and testosterone bottoming out, your coordination and dexterity are taking a dive, too. This means cheerleader pyramids and torch juggling are out. For amateurs at least. Professionals can continue to break their limbs and burn the hair off their scalp at their own risk.

257

Ouchers!

As estrogen nosedives and takes pain-reducing endorphins with it, you're lots more sensitive to aches and pains. And you're pretty sure that itchy sweaters, sheets with less than a 900 thread count, and scratchy, one-ply toilet papers are all the work of the devil.

Energy

If your body was a car, the needle on the gas gauge would be on that big E. And the next gas stop isn't for at least another twenty-four hours, when energizing estrogen and testosterone begin to rise again. Which probably explains that coasting-on-fumes feeling you've got today as your pep and stamina hit rock-bottom levels.

When it comes to sleep, it's a regular princess-and-the-pea situation tonight as bottomed out estrogen has you feeling every little bump on the bed. Even a cookie crumb on your sheet feels as if you are laying on Mount Vesuvius. What's more, you're most sensitive to odors and noise. Even the slightest aroma or sound can awaken you.

Looking for a deeper night's slumber? Pop a pain reliever thirty minutes before bedtime, open a window to air out the bedroom, and mask noise with a fan, air conditioner, a machine that makes those rolling wave sounds, or whatever else you got. And if a noradrenaline burst wakes you up in the middle of the night, do something really boring till you fall back asleep, like counting sheep. Or reading the Olsen twins biography.

Diet

With progesterone so low, cravings are much weaker. But with premenstrual aches and pains high, you still may be tempted to self-medicate with comfort foods. Go with it. By tomorrow you'll be eating 12 percent less anyway.

Continue eating fibrous foods and noshing every three or four hours. Progesterone has a lesser effect today. But even its slight amount can affect disrupt normal digestion and blood sugar.

Cramp alert!

Take ibuprofen (such as Advil or Motrin) today. This will prevent the development of prostaglandins—hormone-like substances that cause the inflammation and pain of menstrual cramps. The result? On Day 1, you'll experience fewer cramps—or even prevent cramps from occurring altogether!

Endnotes

Introduction

1. There are hundreds of hormones in the human body, each with its own function. This book deals with three of the most powerful hormones affecting menstruating women: estrogen, testosterone, and progesterone.

2. Psychologist David Wechsler, Ph.D., who created IQ tests that eliminated sexual bias, found that, when it comes to solving maze puzzles, men scored 92 percent versus women's 8 percent, regardless of culture.

3. Research by Berte Pakkenberg, M.D., a neurologist at Copenhagen Municipal Hospital, shows that woman tend to score about three percent higher on intelligence tests than men.

4. Research by Raquel Gur, M.D., and Ruben Gur, Ph.D., at the University of Pennsylvania shows that women have more gray matter than men. Women also have more extensive connections between neurons and between the two halves of the brain than men. Wechsler's research shows that women's verbal abilities are superior to men.

5. Drs. Gur found that men lose brain tissue at nearly three times the rate of women as they age from their late teens until their mid-forties. Additional research shows that women are more sensitive than men to facial expressions; women have better verbal and nonverbal memories than men; women perform finely coordinated movements better than men; and women can repeat tongue twisters more fluently and accurately than men. Marianne J. Legato, M.D., *Eve's Rib* (New York: Harmony Books, 2002), 26–27.

6. Men make ten times as much testosterone than women. Men make estrogen, but women make ten times more. Michael

Smolensky, Ph.D., and Lynne Lamberg, *The Body Clock Guide to Better Health* (New York: Henry Holt and Company, 2000), 124.

7. In men, testosterone comes in five to seven waves a day. It's highest in the morning and lowest in the evening. Barbara Pease and Allen Pease, *Why Men Don't Listen and Women Can't Read Maps* (New York: Welcome Rain Publishers, 2000), 198.

Day 1

1. Estrogen is an umbrella term that refers to all types of estrogens in the body. Each estrogen serves a different purpose at different stages of a woman's life. During your menstruating years, it's the estrogen "estradiol" that's most potent. For the sake of simplicity, and because most women are more familiar with the term estrogen than estradiol, I chose to use the term estrogen throughout the book.

2. Estrogen is one of the declining hormones that causes withdrawal symptoms contributing to PMS. Once estrogen begins to rise in your body, estrogen withdrawal stops and the positive aspects of rising estrogen and testosterone begin. Deborah Sichel, M.D., and Jeanne Watson Driscoll, M.S., R.N., C.N., *Women's Moods* (New York: Quill, 1999), 84; Elizabeth Lee Vliet, M.D., *Screaming to Be Heard* (New York: M. Evans and Company, Inc., 2001), 68.

3. As estrogen rises, it causes the brain chemicals serotonin, dopamine, and endorphins to increase. These chemicals elevate mood and produce feelings of happiness and contentment. Sichel and Driscoll, 51, 82.

4. While the amount of testosterone your body *produces* daily doesn't fluctuate throughout your menstrual cycle, the amount your brain *uses* depends directly on your estrogen level. That's because estrogen creates testosterone receptors in the brain. And without these receptors, testosterone can't attach to your brain. So the more estrogen you have, the more testosterone influences you. Vliet, 82.

5. More women in the premenstrual and menstrual phases of their cycle preferred comedies and other humorous TV programs than women in the middle of their cycle. The researchers speculate that women might use humorous shows to distract themselves from physical discomfort and to boost their mood. Jeanne Meadowcroft and Dolf Zillmann, "Women's comedy preferences during the menstrual cycle," *Communication Research* 14 (1987): 204–218.

6. There are many studies that show how estrogen affects brain function. In one study, researchers discovered that the nerve cells in rats' brains "grow in complexity" when exposed to estrogen. This increases the connections among nerve cells in an area of the brain needed to store new memories, retrieve older ones, and recall the location of an object or event in space. The researchers speculate the same effect on nerve cells is true for humans. Vladimir Znamensky et al., "Estrogen Levels Regulate the Subcellular Distribution of Phosphorylated Akt in Hippocampal CA1 Dendrites," *The Journal of Neuroscience* 23 (March 15, 2003): 6, 2340.

   There are many studies that show how testosterone affects brain function. One such study suggests that giving women even a single dose of testosterone improves the ability to recall the location of objects. Albert Postma et al., "Effects of testosterone administration on selective aspects of object-location memory in healthy young women," *Psychoneuroendocrinology* 25 (2000): 6, 563–575 (13).

7. Several studies show that estrogen treatment enables menopausal women to make decisions more accurately and with greater confidence. Edward L. Klaiber, M.D., *Hormones and the Mind* (New York: Quill, 2002), 22. Indecision is a symptom of diminished testosterone. Uzzi Reiss, M.D./O.B. G.Y.N., *Natural Hormone Balance* (New York: Pocket Books, 2001), 166.

8. Pakkenberg. Gur and Gur. Wechsler.

9. According to a study by Kathryn Hood, Ph.D., women initiate more conversations midcycle than during their premenstrual or menstrual phases. Kathryn E. Hood, "Contextual determinants of menstrual cycle effects in observations of social interactions," Menstrual Health in Women's Lives (Urbana-Chicago: University of Illinois Press, 1992), 83–97. In Hood's 1992 study, she found that women experience a "menstrual quietude" around their premenstrual and menstrual phases. During this time, women have less interest in going out and socializing, they seek peace and quiet, and they're more contemplative.

10. According to research by Paul Zak, Ph.D., Claremont Graduate University.

11. Your testosterone level affects how many sexually charged dreams and fantasies you have. Klaiber, 107.

12. Your testosterone level affects sexual desire, arousability in your nipples, and clitoris and libido. It also affects how intense your

orgams are. When testosterone is high, orgasms are intense and felt all over your body. When testosterone is low, orgasms are diminished in intensity and feel localized. Klaiber, 107.

13. While estrogen affects lubrication, it does not appear to contribute to sex drive or desire. Gale Malesky et al., *The Hormone Connection* (New York: Rodale, 2001), 128–129.

14. Orgasms help alleviate menstrual cramps and studies have also shown that a woman's pain threshold increases substantially during orgasm. Michael Seeber, Carin Gorrell, Michael Ross, "His & hers . . . and how to have them," *Psychology Today*, 34 (November-December, 2001): 6, 48.

15. A survey of more than 2,000 women at Yale University shows that women who exclusively used tampons, or who were at least sometimes sexually active during their periods, were less likely to have endometriosis. Erika L. Meaddough, etal., "Sexual Activity, Orgasm and *Tampon* Use Are Associated with a Decreased Risk for Endometriosis," *Gynecologic and Obstetric Investigation* 53 (2002): 3, 163–169.

16. Researchers at Rutgers University believe the same chemical that causes the orgasm sensation in the brain (the vasoactive intestinal peptide) may also have strong pain-suppressing qualities rivaling morphine that one day may make it a natural source of pain relief. B. R. Komisaruk et al., "Neural Mechanisms of genital stimulation-produced pain blockage in females," The Conference on Gender and Pain at the National Institutes of Health, Bethesda, Maryland Session, 5, April 8, 1998.

17. Testosterone is known to make both men and women impulsive. And those with higher levels are usually "single, aggressive, and dominate and take risks." Brock Smith, R.Ph., "Testosterone and Its Benefit to Women," ProjectAWARE, *www.project-aware.org/Resource/articlearchives/testosterone.shtml*.

18. Canadian researchers who studied data on menstruating women aged eighteen to sixty-four from the 1999 National Health Interview Survey found that only about 63 percent of women with a heavier than normal menstrual flow make it in to work, whereas 73.5 percent of women with a low or normal menstrual flow make it in to work.

19. N. Milman, J. Clausen, and K. E. Byg, "Iron status in 268 Danish women aged 18–30 years: influence of menstruation, contraceptive method, and iron supplementation," *Annals of Hematology* 77 (August 1998): 1–2, 13–19.

20. L. Rossander, L. Hallberg, and Bjorn-Rasmussen, "E. Absorption of iron from breakfast meals," *American Journal of Clinical Nutrition* 32 (December 1979): 2484–2489.

21. Numerous studies point to a direct connection between menstruation and a heightened desire for comfort foods. For instance, according to one nutrition expert, Maria Karalis, R.D., during stressful times, your body often craves carbohydrates because stress causes your body to break down feel-good serotonin. Eating foods high in carbohydrates triggers the body to release insulin, which then prompts the brain to produce serotonin. Maria Karalis, R.D., "Why We Crave Comfort Foods?," *iKidney, www. ikidney.com/iKidney/Lifestyles/NutritionalTips/JustDiagnosed/ WhyWeCraveComfortFoods.htm*. With all the aches and pains that come with bottoming out estrogen, menstruation is usually a stressful experience on some level for most women.

    Additionally, with testosterone low, you're not taking many risks. So you're less likely to want to try new or exotic foods.

22. A Tufts University study shows that progesterone increases appetite by 12 percent. Vliet, 36.

23. You're hungry more often in the second half of your cycle because of progesterone, which prompts you to eat more so your body can sustain a pregnancy. Vliet, 36.

24. During the second half of your cycle, progesterone boosts your cravings. In one study, 74.3 percent of the women studied reported at least mild food cravings during PMS compared to 56.3 percent during menstruation and 26.9 percent postmenstrually. L. Dye, P. Warner, and J. Bancroft, "Food craving during the menstrual cycle and its relationship to stress, happiness of relationship and depression: A preliminary study," *Journal of Affective Disorders* 34 (1995): 157–164.

    Other research shows that the women report specific cravings for sweets, carbohydrates, fats, and salty foods because of a decrease in serotonin, which occurs when estrogen declines. These foods boost serotonin. Terry Mason, "The PMS and Food Connection," *Health A to Z, www.healthatoz.com/healthatoz/Atoz/ hc/wom/fitn/alert09112001.html*.

25. A brain scan study of normal, hungry people conducted by Gene-Jack Wang, M.D., of Brookhaven National Laboratory showed their brains lit up when they saw and smelled their favorite foods in much the same way as the brains of cocaine addicts when they

think about their next snort. Gene-Jack Wang, M.D., et al., "Exposure to appetitive food stimuli markedly activates the human brain," *NeuroImage* 21 (April 2004): 4, 1790–1797.

26. Water retention and swollen breasts are caused by progesterone because these help the body prepare for a growing fetus. Another effect of progesterone is to slow down the movement of food through the gastrointestinal tract so more nutrients will be absorbed into your bloodstream. The downside is that you hold more in the intestine, making you feel bloated.

27. Many chronic illnesses flare around the time of menstruation. Smolensky and Lamberg, 11. Women who suffer from irritable bowel syndrome often experience a worsening in symptoms during their periods. L. A. Houghton, R. Lea, N Jackson, and P. J. Whorwell, "The menstrual cycle affects rectal sensitivity in patients with irritable bowel syndrome but not healthy volunteers," *Gut* 50 (April 2002): 471–474. According to studies by Margie Profet, Ph.D., women have fewer onsets and contractions of colds and flu during menses.

28. K. Perkins, M. Levine, and M. Marcus, "Tobacco withdrawal in women and menstrual cycle phase," *Journal of Consulting and Clinical Psychology* 68 (2000): 1, 176–80.

29. Legato, 66.

30. Three out of four adults admitted to hospitals for treatment of life-threatening asthma attacks are women, and hospital admissions occur four times more often just before or after menstruation than at any other time of the month. Smolensky and Lamberg, 11.

31. Legato, 186.

32. Migraine researchers have found that certain specific foods such as chocolate, citrus fruits, cheese, and alcohol, especially red wine, can trigger migraine. Migraine Action Association, "What Causes Migraine?," *www.migraine.org.uk/whatcauses.htm*.

33. One of the symptoms of low testosterone is loss of coordination and balance. Reiss, 166.

34. Testosterone speeds up "automatized" behaviors. These are "non-thinking" tasks, such as walking, typing, and scooting out of the way of a table or falling dish. Pierce J. Howard, Ph.D., *The Owner's Manual for the Brain* (Atlanta: Bard Press, 2000), 242.

35. Researchers at Ruhr-Universitat in Bochum, Germany, discovered that a woman's spatial ability (which includes the ability to

read maps, judge distances, and recognize rotated versions of a figure) increases during her period. They believe it's because the low level of estrogen puts the accent on a woman's testosterone, a hormone known for boosting these spatial abilities. Markus Hausmann, *Behavioral Neuroscience* (2000):114, 1245–1250.

36. Estrogen has a direct effect on pain. The more estrogen you have, the less pain you feel; the less estrogen you have, the more pain you feel. Jon-Kar Zubieta, et al., "Regional Mu Opioid Receptor Regulation of Sensory and Affective Dimensions of Pain," *Science* (13 July 2001): 293, 311–315.

37. There have been numerous studies that show a connection between vitamin and mineral supplements and easing of PMS symptoms. Many have been shown to have some benefit. Just a sampling of these studies include the following: A study conducted at Metropolitan Hospital in New York City found that a daily supplement of 1,000 milligrams of calcium reduced premenstrual symptoms in 73 percent of the women who took it. In an Italian study, 360 milligrams of magnesium was associated with fewer cramps, less water retention, and an overall improvement in premenstrual symptoms. Studies show that 400 IUs of vitamin E has been shown to reduce PMS symptoms. Another study by Guy Abraham, M.D., shows 500 milligrams of B_6 a day reduces PMS symptoms.

38. Numerous studies show that taking nonsteroidal anti-inflammatory drugs (NSAIDs), such as ibuprofen, before cramps begin can help lessen or prevent cramps. That's because NSAIDs prevent the production of prostaglandins, chemicals that cause inflammation and trigger transmission of pain signals to the brain. While associated with many types of pains—such as migraine and arthritis—prostaglandins are also the cause of the pain from cramps. However, because NSAIDS are associated with a risk of gastrointestinal bleeding, health experts caution to use these drugs cautiously and according to directions. Eva Martin, M.D., "Menstrual Cramps," *Discovery Health*, *http://health.discovery.com/encyclopedias/2009.html*.

Day 2

1. A 2003 study at the University of Vienna led by psychologist Andreas Mittermair, Ph.D., found that after women drink alcohol, they don't find men more attractive. In fact, the rates of attractiveness actually decreased! "No beer goggles for women?," *Realbeer*, September 23, 2003, *www.realbeer.com/news/articles/news-002035.php*.

2. Researchers at Northwestern University Medical School found that a chemical in red wine believed to help reduce the risk of heart disease is actually a form of estrogen. The substance, resveratrol, is highly concentrated in the skin of grapes and is abundant in red wine. Barry D. Gehm, "Resveratrol, a polyphenolic compound found in grapes and wine, is an antagonist for the estrogen receptor," *Proceedings of the National Academy of Sciences, USA* 94 (December 1997): 14138–14143.

   In a study of women between the ages of eighteen and thirty-five, researchers found that even a small amount of alcohol can quickly increase a woman's level of testosterone, leading to an increased sex drive. Maria Burke, "Real Men Don't Drink," *NewScientist.com*, November 27, 1999, *www.newscientist.com/hottopics/alcohol/alcohol.jsp?id=22145200*.

Day 3

1. According to the results of one study conducted at Brigham and Women's Hospital in Boston, women who consume at least 500 milligrams of caffeine daily, the equivalent of four or five cups of coffee, have nearly 70 percent more estrogen during the early follicular phase (Days 1 to 5) than women consuming no more than 100 milligrams of caffeine daily, or less than one cup of coffee. Daniel W. Cramer, *Fertility and Sterility* (October 2001): 76, 723–729.

Day 4

1. This refers to Hood's 1992 study where she found women have less interest in socializing, they seek out solitude and are more contemplative during PMS and menstruation. When you come out of this phase, the presumption is that you become more interested in socializing and the outer world. And research backs this up. Alexandra Pope, a psychotherapist and author of *The Wild Genie: The Healing Power of Menstruation* (Bowral, Australia: Sally Milner Publishing, 2001) maintains that during the first half of

the cycle, when estrogen rises, women are "more outer focused, linear, left brain, feeling fairly clear (no messy emotion) and productive, with plenty of energy for others." During the second half of the menstrual cycle, when estrogen declines, women "tend to become more inner focused." Alexandra Pope, "Menstruation is Power," Museum of Menstruation, *www.mum.org/menstpow.htm*.

2. Researchers speculate this hormone surges as a way to help you triumph over your rivals since it increases your willingness to take risks, improves reaction time, dexterity, and coordination, and enhances your ability to think fast on your feet. Deborah Blum, *Sex on the Brain* (New York: Penguin Books, 1997), 168, 171. That it also increases libido is simply a delicious bonus. H. S. Bateup et al., "Testosterone, Cortisol, and Women's Competition," *Evolution and Human Behavior*, 3 (November 2002): 23, 181–192.

Day 5

1. A rise in estrogen has been associated with a rise in left hemisphere activity (such as logic and verbal fluency) and a decline in right hemisphere activity (such as creativity and visual-spatial ability, for instance, drawing a three-dimensional object, or reading a map). Northrup, 105.

2. Women have specific areas for speech and language on both sides of the brain. In men, speech and language are primarily in the left brain and have no specific location. This is one reason talking doesn't come as naturally or as easily. Pease and Pease, 70.

3. Testosterone is a hormone that pumps up your assertiveness. In fact, it's been reported that British gynecologist Malcolm Whitehead, M.D., claims he prescribed testosterone to a number of female politicians. Bernard Mallee, "Who's on the testosterone? Women trying to survive in the macho world of politics are resorting to hormonal help," *New Statesman* 16 (July 7, 2003): 764, 22.

4. H. S. Bateup, et al., "Testosterone, Cortisol, and Women's Competition," 181–192.

5. Many chronic illnesses flare around the time of menstruation. Smolensky and Lamberg, 11. This is because estrogen is so low. But as it rises, the flare-ups recede.

6. Breast tissue is less dense in the first two weeks of the cycle in premenopausal women, making a mammogram easier to read.

One study of 2,500 women conducted at the Fred Hutchinson Cancer Research Center in Seattle found that women who wait until two weeks after they start their period have the best chance of getting a more accurate reading.

Day 6

1. This refers to the increased estrogen levels giving rise to left hemisphere activity (Northrup, 105) as well as Alexandra Pope's assertion that women tend to become more outwardly focused, linear, and left brained as estrogen rises ("Menstruation is Power").

2. Day 6 to 10 is the time to be bold and make big decisions. Gale Malesky et al., 31.

3. Research shows that the testosterone levels of married men increase along with the testosterone in their wives. Patricia Allen, *Cycles* (New York: Pinnacle Books, 1983), 2.

4. In men, testosterone comes in five to seven waves a day. It's highest in the morning and lowest in the evening. Pease and Pease, 198.

5. Women talk more out loud and verbalize more on high estrogen days. Pease and Pease, 79.

6. Pease and Pease, 96.

7. Studies constantly show that, in business, a woman with a deeper voice is considered more intelligent, authoritative, and credible. Pease and Pease, 96.

8. Also, avoid speaking more loudly. It's a mistake many women make to sound more authoritative. It gives the impression that you're aggressive. Pease and Pease, 96.

Day 7

1. When a woman experiences something unpleasant, estrogen intensifies and prolongs her body's stress response. Research has even found that, when young men are given estrogen, their body's stress response intensifies and becomes prolonged, too. Legato, 40. Researchers at Rockefeller University led by Donald W. Pfaff, Ph.D., found that estrogen increases response to stimuli and "arousal" from stimuli.

2. This refers to the Meadowcroft and Zillman study that found that women prefer comedies during premenstrual and menstrual phases and that left-brained women are more outwardly focused. The presumption is that women prefer less comedy

and more news about the world around them.

3. Rising testosterone pumps up feeling of independence in both women and men. One Harvard study shows that the testosterone levels of husbands and fathers are lower than men who are single and researchers speculate that this decreases a man's urge to wander. Peter B. Gray et al., "Marriage and fatherhood are associated with lower testosterone in males," *Evolution and Human Behavior* 3 (2002): 23, 193–201. Testosterone also pumps up feelings of safety and security. Reiss, 166. This presumably makes you feel more comfortable doing activities alone.

4. According to research by Theresa Crenshaw, M.D., author of *The Alchemy of Love and Lust* (New York: Pocket 1997), when testosterone is high in women, they're more orgasm-driven and reluctant to commit.

5. The Susan G. Komen Breast Cancer Foundation, Resource Guide, *www.ockomen.com/resource_guide/rgearlydetectionstep1.shtml*.

Day 8

1. In a study conducted by scientists at the University of Pennsylvania and the Monell Chemical Senses Center in Philadelphia, women rated their moods for six hours after sniffing male perspiration. The findings suggested something in men's perspiration brightened their moods and relaxed them. George Preti, et al, "Male Axillary Extracts Contain Pheromones that Affect Pulsatile Secretion of Luteinizing Hormone and Mood in Women Recipients" *Biology of Reproduction* 68 (June 2003): 2107–2113.

2. Smolensky and Lamberg, 122.

3. Pease and Pease, 204.

4. Pease and Pease, 204.

Day 9

1. Monthly surges of testosterone boost your sense of personal power. Brock Smith, R.Ph., "Testosterone and Its Benefit to Women." Project-Aware.org, March 2002, *www.project-aware.org/Resource/articlearchives/testosterone.shtml*.

2. Numerous studies show that stress makes your muscles tight, which, in a vicious cycle, intensifies stress. One such study was conducted at Arizona State University in 1992 and examined the effects of a daily ten-minute neck and shoulder massage for twenty-three critical care nurses for a six-week period.

The results revealed that massage is more effective than rest at reducing stress.

3. David M. Buss, Ph.D., author of *The Evolution of Desire*, conducted a global survey of more than 10,000 people in thirty-seven cultures and found it to be universally true that women prefer confident, ambitious, and successful men with money, resources, power, and high social status. In other words, men who have the resources to invest in them and their children.

4. Bernard Mallee, "Who's on the testosterone? Women trying to survive in the macho world of politics are resorting to hormonal help," 22.

Day 10

1. Maria Hernandez-Reif Ph.D., et al, "High blood pressure and associated symptoms were reduced by massage therapy," *Journal of Bodywork and Movement Therapies*, 4 (January 2000): 1, 31–38. Birger Kaada and Ove Torsteinb, "Increase of Plasma Beta Endorphins in a Connective Tissue Massage," *General Pharmacology*, 20 (1989): 4, 487–489.

2. A study conducted by Jill B. Becker, Ph.D., reveals that women are more likely to get addicted to nicotine, cocaine, and other addictive substances if they start the habit at a high-estrogen time of month, due to the way estrogen influences the amount of dopamine released in response to addictive substances. Jill B. Becker et al., "Gender Differences in the Behavioral Responses to Cocaine and Amphetamine: Implications for Mechanisms Mediating Gender Differences in Drug Abuse," *Annals of the New York Academy of Sciences* 937 (June 2001): 172–187.

3. Studies show that women are more apt to flirt as ovulation nears.

4. Studies at the Kinsey Institute for Sex, Gender, and Reproduction show that during sex a man's perception of a woman's attractiveness is related to the depth of his intimate feelings for her. If he doesn't care for her, he sees her as less attractive, even if she's considered physically attractive by others. Pease and Pease, 231.

5. Malesky et al., 31.

Day 11

1. High estrogen has been connected with high confidence. In a study by Rosemarie Krug, a psychophysiologist at the University of Bamberg, women with peaking estrogen were confident in their abilities, unusually quick to come up with solutions on problem-solving tests, and also reluctant to depend on others for help. Blum, 205.

2. You've probably noticed this difference in vision when looking for a lost item. He can look around for hours and not spot it. You can find it in a second. Your wider peripheral vision allows you to scan a wider area than a man can. Pease and Pease, 21.

3. The Kinsey Institute found that 76 percent of men said they wanted sex with the lights on, compared to only 36 percent of women. Pease and Pease, 220.

4. The mere sight of a naked woman is enough to arouse most heterosexual men, whereas a woman needs to use more senses than only sight to become aroused. Pease and Pease, 220.

5. Men prefer women with curves—wide hips, narrow waists, long legs, and round chests. Pease and Pease, 232.

6. Women are capable of seeing greater detail than men. Partly because women's eyes have a greater variety of cones in the retina that allow them to see more shades of color and because of their wider peripheral vision. And partly because, just as most female mammals, women have more finely tuned senses than men. This is because they evolved having to defend their children, while the men were away hunting, and needed to be able to pick up on subtle danger signals. Pease and Pease, 20.

Day 12

1. Jon-Kar Zubieta et al., "Regional Mu Opioid Receptor Regulation of Sensory and Affective Dimensions of Pain," 311–315.

2. Men married to women who are not taking birth-control pills initiate sex about 30 percent more often near the women's ovulation than at other times of the month. Scientists suspect men get clued in to when the time is right because of the pheremones women emit that send the male brain a powerful come-hither message. Smolensky and Lamberg, 122.

3. To show they're listening, men grunt by using short "hmmp's" with an occasional slight nod of the head. They also speak in a more monotone way because they find it harder to decode

the subtle meanings behind higher and lower voice tones that women tend to use. Pease and Pease, 95.

Day 13

1. Scientists at the Columbia College of Physicians and Surgeons in New York have found that breathing in the scent of coconut lowers your heart rate and reduces your level of stress. Carol Krucoff, "Is Your House Making You Fat?," Prevention.com, 2002, *http://msn.prevention.com/cda/feature2002/0,2479,s2-6269,00.html*.

2. Planned Parenthood, "The Facts of Life: A Guide for Teens and Their Families, How Pregnancy Happens," May 2004, *www.plannedparenthood.org/teens/teentalk3.html*.

3. High voices are related to high estrogen levels. Pease and Pease, 96.

4. Pease and Pease, 96.

5. According to research by Mark A. Bellis and R. Robin Baker, women are more likely to have intercourse during ovulation with their lover but not with their husband. R. Robin Baker, Mark A. Bellis, *Human Sperm Competition: Copulation, Masturbation and Infidelity.* (London: Chapman & Hall, 1995)

6. A strong jawline indicates high testosterone, which, in turn, indicates a stronger immune system. Geoffrey Cowley, "The biology of beauty," *Newsweek* 127 (June 3, 1996): 23, 60.

7. When a woman is ovulating or ready to conceive, she's likely to prefer men with more masculine features. When a woman is menstruating, or least likely to get pregnant, she's more likely to prefer softer, more feminine features. David Perrett, et al, "Menstrual Cycle Alters Face Preference," *Nature* 399 (June 24, 1999): 741–742.

8. David Perrett et al., "Menstrual Cycle Alters Face Preference."

9. Pease and Pease, 96.

10. Pease and Pease, 96.

11. C. Wedekind and S. Füri, "Body odour preferences in men and women: do they aim for specific MHC-combinations or simply heterozygosity?," *Proceedings of the Royal Society-Series B* 264 (October 22,1997) 1387: 1471–1479.

12. Pease and Pease, 160.

13. C. Wedekind and S. Füri, "Body odour preferences in men and women: do they aim for specific MHC-combinations or simply heterozygosity?"

14. In a study conducted by Rosemarie King, a psychophysiologist at the University of Bamberg, in Germany, when estrogen peaked, women were turned off when a man acted like a lousy potential father. Blum, 207.

15. Oxytocin is a hormone that boosts how bonded we feel to others. Oxytocin jumps to five times its normal level during climax. Michael Seeber, Carin Gorrell, Michael Ross, "His & hers . . . and how to have them," *Psychology Today* 34 (November-December, 2001): 6, 48.

16. Mark A. Bellis and R. Robin Baker, "Do females promote sperm competition? Data for humans," *Animal Behaviour* 40 (1990): 997–999.

17. Sexual desire and fantasies peak around ovulation, as well as intensity of orgasm. Smolensky and Lamberg, 122.

18. Smolensky and Lamberg, 11.

Day 14

1. Smolensky and Lamberg, 126. Allen, 14.

2. There are not one, but two estrogen drops and, therefore, withdrawal phases in each menstrual cycle. Each plunge in estrogen creates an estrogen withdrawal state as this hormone unbinds from the estrogen receptors in the brain. Sichel and Driscoll, 82.

3. Numerous studies and experts report that declining progesterone produces withdrawal symptoms. One such study was conducted by Sheryl S. Smith, Ph.D., at Allegheny University of the Health Sciences and was titled "GABA Receptor Alpha-4 Subunit Suppression Prevents Withdrawal Properties of an Endogenous Steroid." This study shows that postpartum depression and PMS share a common cause: the withdrawal of a sedative molecule found in progesterone. Richard Karel, "PMS, Postpartum Depression, Sedative Withdrawal Believed to Have Common Brain-Receptor Link," Psychiatric News, May 15, 1998, *www.psych.org/pnews/98-05-15/link.html*.

4. There are numerous studies supporting the idea that hormone withdrawal is the cause of PMS and what this book introduces as pre-PMS. Smith's study is one that supports the idea of progesterone withdrawal symptoms. Experts including Sichel and Driscoll report that declining estrogen results in withdrawal symptoms. Sichel and Driscoll, 82. Studies and experts point to side effects of declining testosterone. Reiss, 166. And one study even points to a syndrome that occurs in men when testosterone declines, which presumably would also happen in women when testosterone

declines. G. A. Lincoln, "The irritable male syndrome," *Reproductive Fertility Development* 13 (2001):7–8, 567–76.

5. As you probably already know, the intensity of pre-PMS and PMS varies in intensity from woman to woman. Researchers speculate that it may be because some women are born with an increased biological vulnerability to shifting hormones. This causes the receptors and cells in some women's brains to not be able to withstand the impact of hormonal changes as much as others. Sichel and Driscoll, 51. Malesky et al., 28, 29.

6. Testosterone deficiency in women results in lower self-esteem. Reiss, 166.

7. When estrogen decreases, so does the feel-good brain chemical serotonin. Low serotonin is often related to depression. Sichel and Driscoll, 82.

8. Blum, 179.

9. According to April 2004 research by sociologist Werner Habermehl from the Hamburg Medical Research Institute.

10. During the second half of your menstrual cycle, you become reflective, cut down on social activities and going out, and become more conscious of what's not working in your life. Christiane Northrup, M.D., *Women's Bodies, Women's Wisdom* (New York: Bantam, 2002), 110.

11. Decreasing estrogen decreases serotonin, which causes feelings of sadness and insecurity. Sichel and Driscoll, 82.

12. When your serotonin drops, you'll tend to withdraw and become anxious and reclusive. Legato, 13.

13. Research shows that progesterone has a tranquilizing effect on the brain, much like antianxiety medications. Vliet, 37.

14. Some women experience a feeling of soothing calm when progesterone rises. Other women feel depression, fatigue, tiredness, or lethargy when progesterone rises. Vliet, 37.

15. The rise in estrogen levels has been associated with a rise in left hemisphere activity and a decline in right hemisphere activity. Northrup, 105.

16. A 1998 study led by Barbara Fredrickson, Ph.D., at the University of Michigan found that women who felt bad about their body image scored lower in math. B. L. Fredrickson et al., "That swimsuit becomes you: Sex differences in self-objectification, restrained eating, and math performance," Journal of Personality and Social Psychology, 75 (July 1998): 269–284.

17. Howard, 234–235.

18. Pease and Pease, 157.

19. One such marketing expert who endorses using the power of progesterone to sway female shoppers to buy more is Martha Barletta, author of *Marketing to Women: How to Understand, Reach and Increase Your Share of the World's Largest Market* Segment (Chicago: Dearborn Trade, 2002).

20. A deficiency in estrogen and testosterone produce a lack of energy and stamina and daylong fatigue. Reiss, 29, 166.

21. One of the metabolites of progesterone (3-alphaOH-DHP) has been found to be about eight times more potent as a CNS barbiturate known today, methohexital. Vliet, 78.

22. L. Dye, P. Warner, and J. Bancroft, "Food craving during the menstrual cycle and its relationship to stress, happiness of relationship and depression: A preliminary study," *Journal of Affective Disorders* 34 (1995): 157–164.
    Terry Mason, "The PMS and Food Connection," *Health A to Z*, *www.healthatoz.com/healthatoz/Atoz/hc/wom/fitn/alert09112001.jsp*.

23. According to one study, women who were dieting or restricting their food intake reported fewer food cravings than those who were not. I. T. Cohen, B. B. Sherwin, and A. S. Fleming, "Food cravings, mood and the menstrual cycle," *Hormones and Behavior* 21 (1987): 457–470.

24. According to a 1989 study by Robert Thayer, Ph.D., brisk ten-minute walks reduce food cravings and improved mood.

25. Vliet, 36.

26. Progesterone makes your blood sugar fall more rapidly. This makes you feel hungrier more often. Vliet, 36.

27. Allen, 69.

28. One woman in three reports more frequent constipation and hard stools after ovulation. That's because progesterone exerts a constipating effect. Smolensky and Lamberg, 243.

29. Michael Biamonte, C.C.N., "The True Cause of Candida!," The Biomonte Center for Clinical Nutrition, *www.health-truth.com/articles/Candida3.asp*.

30. The rapid drop in estrogen may trigger onset of a migraine in some women. Vliet, 35.

31. According to research conducted by Edward M. Wojtys, M.D., at the University of Michigan in Ann Arbor, women are close to three times as likely to sustain a common knee injury during ovulation than at other points in their menstrual cycle. Edward M.

Wojtys, M.D., et al., "Association Between the Menstrual Cycle and Anterior Cruciate Ligament Injuries in Female Athletes," The American Journal of Sports Medicine, 26 (September-October 1998): 614–619.

32. Allen, 10.

Day 15

1. Progesterone causes a delay in word recall and verbal responses. Vliet, 78.

2. Vliet, 78.

3. Stephen Luntz, "Exercise Enhanced During the Menstrual Cycle," *Australasian Science*, January/February 2003, *www.control.com. au/bi2003/articles241/up5_241.shtml.*

Day 16

1. Women experience a nesting instinct premenstrually. This may result in the urge to nurture your mate, clean, organize, or decorate to make your place more homey. Katherine Elgin, *Twenty-Eight Days* (New York: Random House, 1984), 43.

2. Study after study shows that high estrogen and testosterone lead to better memory, learning ability, verbal ability, and concentration. Whereas, low estrogen and testosterone lead to poorer memory, learning ability, verbal ability, and mental fogginess.

3. Numerous studies point to the preference of curvy bodies over thin ones. According to one such survey conducted by John Krantz, Ph.D., of Hanover University, both men and women choose a moderate, curvy shape over the stick-thin fashion model shape. J. H. Krantz, J. Ballard, and J. Scher, "Comparing the results of laboratory and World-Wide Web Samples on the determinants of female attractiveness," *Behavior Research Methods, Instruments, & Computers* 29 (1997): 264–269.

   Additionally, Barbara Pease and Allen Pease report that men prefer women with softness and curves where they have firmness and flat areas. Men prefer women with wide hips, narrow waists, long legs, and round chests—all attributes they will never possess. Pease and Pease, 232.

4. Devendra Singh, Ph.D., of Cambridge University, surveyed men of numerous nationalities and concluded that men had unconsciously learned sometime in the past that curves signal fertility and health and subsequently had it prewired into their brains.

D. Singh, "Female Mate Value at a Glance: Relationship of Waist-to-Hip Ratio to Health, Fecundity, and Attractiveness," *Neuroendocrinology Letters* Special Issue (2002): 23, 81–91.

5. D. Singh, "Female Mate Value at a Glance: Relationship of Waist-to-Hip Ratio to Health, Fecundity, and Attractiveness," 81–91.

6. D. Singh, "Female Mate Value at a Glance: Relationship of Waist-to-Hip Ratio to Health, Fecundity, and Attractiveness," 81–91.

7. Research shows that it's normal for women to have extra fat on hips and thighs, since these are the spots from which the milk supply is drawn. J. Hoffman, Patrick J. Bird, "Ask the Experts: Biology, Why does fat deposit on the hips and thighs of women and around the stomachs of men?" *Scientific American*, September 23, 2002, *www.sciam.com*.

8. It's generally agreed by health experts that women with more fat on their body have an easier transition to menopause because of the storage of estrogen in their fat cells.

Day 18

1. According to Ann Louise Gittleman, Ph.D., C.N.S., regular table salt is chemically processed, so it doesn't dissolve quickly, which means it can build up and causes bloat. But natural unrefined does not contains chemicals, so it doesn't cause bloat. Anne Louise Gittleman, Ph.D., C.N.S., "Nutrition Know-How," First for Women, (January 5, 2004), 40.

Day 19

1. Up till Day 22, your body prepares for pregnancy in case your womb was fertilized during ovulation. As part of this preparation, progesterone rises to prompt your body to thicken your uterine lining, as well as slow you down and increase your appetite so you'll be more likely to keep your baby safe and eat enough for two. By Day 23, your body knows whether or not your egg was fertilized. If it was, estrogen and progesterone continue to rise. If not, estrogen and progesterone fall.

2. Alexandra Pope, "Menstruation is Power."

3. Michael Seeber, Carin Gorrell, Michael Ross, "His & hers . . . and how to have them," *Psychology Today*, 34 (November-December, 2001): 6, 48.

Day 20

1. Intuition and gut instinct are more pronounced when you're more in touch with your emotions, such as when you're in your right brain phase. And if you ever doubted that a woman's intuition was real, a study by Raquel Gur, M.D., and Ruben Gur, Ph.D., may provide proof. In their study, fMRI brain scans revealed that, when men and women make their minds a blank, a man's brain shows just 30 percent of electrical activity while a woman's brain shows 90 percent of electrical activity. A primary purpose of one of the brain areas that remains active is to filter emotional reactions to the environment. This suggests that women receive and interpret signals from their environment even when at rest, accounting for their "sixth sense." Sichel and Driscoll, 30.

Day 23

1. Based on clinical research by Sichel and Driscoll, the first drop in estrogen after ovulation may sensitize serotonin receptors in the brain and the second drop may exacerbate the reaction. This may be why the symptoms of PMS are more intense than pre-PMS. Sichel and Driscoll, 83.

2. Numerous studies show that caffeine exacerbates PMS. In one such study, women who drank one cup of coffee per day increased their risk of developing PMS by 30 percent. The risk jumped to 700 percent in women who drank eight to ten cups per day. A. Rossignol, H. Bonnlander, "Caffeine-containing beverages, total fluid consumption, and premenstrual syndrome," *American Journal of Public Health* 80 (September, 1990): 9, 1106–1110.

3. Progesterone withdrawal produces effects similar to other medications that act at the GABA receptor, such as benzodiazepines and barbiturates, including increased anxiety, restlessness, insomnia, and tearfulness. Vliet, 78.

4. While it's widely accepted that tears relieve stress, researchers don't agree why. Some believe that tears release feel-good endorphins. William Frey II, Ph.D., a St. Paul, Minnesota, biochemist and tear expert, believes that tears flush stress chemicals out of the body. His research seems to back his conclusion up. In one of his studies, he found that emotional tears have a different chemical makeup than tears that occur from irritation, such as that caused by onion vapors. Judy Foreman, "Sob Story: Why we cry, and how," *Boston Globe* (October 21, 1996): C1.

5. Malesky et al., 31.
6. Numerous studies show that because noradrenaline and sero-tonin are sensitive and respond to your environment and people around you, simple acts of kindness can dramatically reduce noradrenaline's stress effects.
7. "During sex, a woman is acutely aware of outside sounds or environmental changes, but a man is totally focused and undis-tracted. This is a woman's ancient nest-defending biology in action—she is monitoring sounds to make sure nothing is sneak-ing up to steal her offspring." Pease and Pease, 214.
8. Women may be more sensitive to acrid, bad odors—from coffee, benzine, or camphor—twenty-four to forty-eight hours before their period. Walker, 96.
9. Women are capable of seeing greater detail than men, partly because of the difference in their eyes. Women's eyes have a greater variety of cones in the retina that allow them to see more shades of color and have wider peripheral vision. And partly because, as do most female mammals, women have more finely tuned senses than men. This is because they evolved having to defend their children while the men were away hunting, so they needed to be able to pick up on subtle danger signals. Pease and Pease, 20.
10. A drop in estradiol triggers a firing of the "alerting" centers in the brain. These centers then discharge a burst of noradrena-line, which has an arousing effect and wakes you up. Vliet, 232.
11. According to a National Sleep Foundation survey conducted by the Gallup Organization February 27 through March 17, 1996, roughly eight in ten people (83 percent) who had tried non-pre-scription medications specifically for nighttime pain relief said they were very (26 percent) or somewhat (57 percent) effective.
12. Most odors—pleasant or unpleasant—can interrupt sleep. Peter Badia, Ph.D., Michelle Boecher, Ph.D., and Kenneth P. Wright, Jr., "Olfactory Sensitivity in Sleep and the Effects of Fragrances on the Quality of Sleep," Sense of Smell Institute, 1991. During menstruation, sleep is already light, so you're more likely to be woken up by scents.
13. According to research by John Shepard, M.D., medical direc-tor of the Mayo Clinic Sleep Disorders Center, a loud constant noise, such as that produced by a fan or air conditioner, helps you sleep because the brain is designed to sleep best when

surrounded by continuous sound—even if it's loud. It's intermittent sound—such as snoring—that wakes you up. Douglas Lichterman, "Tired of Feeling Tired? Here's How to Get the Sleep You Need," *Woman's World* XXIV (January 21, 2003): 3, 14–15.

14. An American Academy of Sleep Medicine study found that a ten-minute nap improved performance for at least an hour after the subjects were awakened—and was even more energizing than a longer nap! Doug Brunk, "Brief Naps More Recuperative for Sleep Deprived," *Family Pratice News* 30 (Sept 15, 2000): 9.

15. Smolensky and Lamberg, 126, 128.

Day 24

1. In a Masters and Johnson study, some women reported masturbating to orgasm at or just before the onset of menstruation to find relief from pelvic congestion. Allen, 119.
2. Smolensky and Lamberg, 126.
3. Vliet, 236.
4. Chamomile's sedative effect is believed to be attributable to the flavinoid component apigenin, which binds to the same receptors as benzodiazepines. Michael M. Larzelere, Ph.D., and Pamela Wiseman, M.D., "Anxiety, depression, and insomnia," *Primary Care; Clinics in Office Practice* 29 (June 2002): 2.

    Researchers used to believe that the tryptophan in milk made it easier to fall asleep. But later studies show that there's such a scant amount of tryptophan in milk that you'd have to drink a gallon to get the effect. Now they believe that milk simply gives you a fuller feeling, which makes it easier to sleep.

Day 25

1. Comfort food relieves stress and puts you in a great mood, according to a study conducted at the University of California, San Francisco. That's because, as the study shows, sugary and starchy treats puts the brakes on the adrenal hormones that cause stress reactions, making you feel happier. M. F. Dallman *et al.*, "Chronic stress and obesity: A new view of 'comfort food," *Proceedings of the National Academy of Sciences* 100 (September 15, 2003) 20, 11696–11701.
2. Smolensky and Lamberg, 11.

Day 27

1. A menstrual hut is a house where women are segregated from the rest of the community during menstruation. It's a phenomena that's been found in many ancient cultures around the world.

2. You've already been contemplative and slower during the second half of your cycle. This phase refers to an even more stepped up version of what you've been experiencing—low interest in socializing and low interest in doing even simple activities.

3. It's widely accepted by sleep experts that television stimulates the brain, making it harder to fall asleep. Some researchers also believe that the light from TV disrupts your body's production of melatonin, the "sleep hormone" that helps maintain regular sleep cycles.

4. NSAIDS work for up to 75 percent of women with cramps. The trick is to start taking them days before your period comes to combat pain-inducing prostaglandins. It should be noted that there is a risk of gastrointestinal bleeding with NSAIDS. A.D.A.M. Inc., Well-Connected series, *www.healthandage.com*.

Day 28

1. On the last day of your menstrual cycle, your hormones reach the bottom of their cycle. This triggers menstruation.

2. According to research by Scott Haltzman, M.D., your mate wants to please you because it fuels his self-confidence.

3. According to research by Scott Haltzman, M.D., women tend to "hint" at what they want. However, a man's brain isn't wired to pick up on hints as a woman's is. They require concrete, detailed instructions.

We've

conceived

a better way

for you

to conceive.

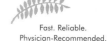

$\mathcal{N}$ow there's an easier
way for you to know when you are
ovulating. It's called the
Ovulation Scope, and it's a true
breakthrough in ovulation testing.
The Ovulation Scope is an ovulation
test that relies on saliva samples,
rather than urine samples. So
it's easier and much more
convenient than previous
over-the-counter
ovulation tests.

The #1

selling

saliva

ovulation

test

available.

Track

your

cycle with the

Ovulation

Scope.

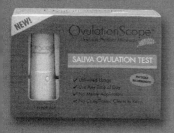

OvulationScope™
Ovulation Predictor Microscope

Your test just got easier.

www.ovulationscope.com

Available at Target & Walmart

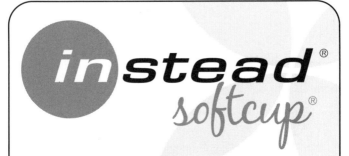
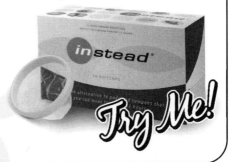